Intermittent Fasting and Weight Loss for Women – 2 Books in 1

The Only Guide You Need to Lose Weight Fast and Keep It Off for Good!

Learn How to Slow Aging and Feel More Attractive in 3 Weeks!

By

Nancy Johson

Nancy Johnson

Weight Loss for Women

The Ultimate Guide for Women to Lose Weight, Burn Fat, Reset their Metabolism, Stop Aging and Live Longer!

By

Nancy Johnson

Nancy Johnson

render any resulting actions solely under their purview. There are no scenarios in which the publisher or the original author of this work can be in any fashion deemed liable for any hardship or damages that may befall them after undertaking information described herein.

Additionally, the information in the following pages is intended only for informational purposes and should thus be thought of as universal. As befitting its nature, it is presented without assurance regarding its prolonged validity or interim quality. Trademarks that are mentioned are done without written consent and can in no way be considered an endorsement from the trademark holder.

Table of Contents

Nancy Johnson

Introduction

Most women over 50 feel as if they have lost their ability to be attractive, healthy and feel good in their own bodies. But what is the cause for this widespread issue? The fact is that in today's world we are spending more and more time at home and we have significantly reduced our need for food. However, even if we do not need as many calories as we did in the past to survive and be healthy, most of us are still eating as if they were running a marathon a day.

Therefore, it should not come as a surprise that most women over 50 years of age are out of shape, overweight and unhealthy. This normally translates into a worse quality of life and is something that is frustrating for a substantial portion of the female population. Thanks to researches and scientific studies conducted by incredible nutritionists, it is now possible to overcome the negative effect of a sedentary life. In fact, intermittent fasting seems like the perfect solution for all those women that want to burn fat, lose weight and gain a healthy and new lifestyle.

The need of all these women is what inspired the writing of this guide. In fact, in the next chapters you are not going to find complicated explanations of scientific topics that, even if interesting, do not give you a clear direction on what you can do to start feeling better. On the contrary, while writing this book, a great effort was made to make sure that each concept is followed by a subsequent strategy that can be implemented in a healthy intermittent fasting protocol.

By reading this book you will get all the information and practical steps you need to follow to start intermittent fasting in just a few days. We advise you to talk to your doctor before changing your diet as intermittent fasting is not suitable if you have certain healthy conditions.

Please, be aware that the goal of this book is to give you accurate information on intermittent fasting, but it does not take the place of a true medical advice. We hope that you can find motivational and informative insights that help you make a change for the better.

Chapter 1 - The most Important Component: Mindset

One of the most important tools at your disposal when you decide to lose weight and win a healthier lifestyle is your ability to make long lasting changes to your routine. In order to do this, you need to have a positive and effective mindset that can sustain you when things get difficult. That is why we have decided to dedicate the first few chapters of this book to this extremely important topic.

The willpower, also known as self-discipline, self-control or determination, is the ability to control your behaviors, emotions and focus. The willpower involves the ability to resist impulses and sacrifice immediate gratification in order to achieve your goals. It also includes the ability to ignore unwelcome thoughts, feelings or impulses, as well as that of self-regulation. The level of willingness of a woman can determine its ability to save for its financial stability, to make positive choices for its mental and physical health and to avoid the use or abuse of harmful substances. Continuing to give up instant gratifications in favor of future prizes, you can move towards your goals and develop your willpower. Thanks to a constant "workout" of the mind, this practice will strengthen your ability to control your impulses, exactly how physical exercise strengthens your muscles.

Let's take a look at some tips that can help you build up your mindset.

Evaluate your habits

If you are trying to improve your willpower, probably your inability to control your impulses is negatively affecting some areas of your life. Some women over 50 struggle with their willpower in every aspect of their life, while others are limited to having some specific "weaknesses". Determine what the area you intend to improve and, if the areas are a lot, choose to dedicate yourself to one at a time.

For example, your willpower could be weak in front of the food. This could consequently negatively affect your health and quality of your life For example, you may have difficulty following your intermittent fasting protocol, which causes you to binge and not be healthy. Whatever health issue you are facing today, acknowledging it is the first step to overcome it.

Create a scale to evaluate your willpower

You will need to evaluate your willpower as efficiently as possible during your intermittent fasting protocol. You could create a scale from 1 to 10, in which 1 represents a complete indulgence relative to the thing, or to things, that you are trying to avoid, and 10 a stoic respect for the restrictive rules that you have established for yourself. Alternatively you can develop a simpler scale, based on "at all, little, more, much". This scale can take different forms, while continuing to offer you the opportunity to evaluate yourself while following an intermittent fasting protocol.

For example, if you realize you eat sweets in a compulsive way or stop in some fast food restaurants on a daily basis, on a scale from 1 to 10 you can evaluate yourself with a 1 or a 2.

Think long term

If you want to improve yourself, the first step to take is to set a goal for your change. You will need to choose a clear, specific and achievable goal. If it were too vague or not measurable, it would indeed be difficult to determine any progress made or establish it achieved.

For example, the "eating healthier" goal, established by those women who tend to eat impulsively, will certainly be too vague. "Healthier" is a relative concept, which will make it difficult to establish when it was reached. A more concrete destination could be to "lose 20 pounds through a healthy intermittent fasting protocol", "return to a size 44" or "overcoming my sugar addiction ".

Have short term goals as well

When you want to reach an important goal (which could appear complicated), one of the best ways to do this is to establish intermediate goals along the way. Your short-term goals must also be specific and measurable, and able to lead you to your final goal.

For example, if you are trying to lose 20 pounds, you can give you a first short-term goal similar to "losing 5 pounds", "do exercise 3 times a week" or "limit desserts to once a week".

Think big

The best way to "train" your willpower is to show you are willing to sacrifice the desire for immediate gratification in favor of a better long-term reward. The final compensation will be that of "living well" or "feeling attractive"; However, to learn how to exercise your willpower it is advisable to establish a concrete prize.

For example, if your desire is to lose weight, trying to control your compulsive hunger through a healthy intermittent fasting protocol, your final reward could be a new dress that makes you feel amazing.

Give up immediate gratification

This is the essence of the development of willpower. When you feel tempted to give up to an impulse, realize that what you really want to live is that short feeling of immediate gratification. In case your impulsive behavior is contrary to your goals, after giving away to immediate gratification you will feel guilty.

To resist the desire for immediate gratification, follow these steps.

- Recognize what you want to do.
- Admit that the only thing you want is immediate gratification.
- Remember your short and long-term goals you set for yourself.
- Ask yourself if it's worth giving to the current impetus and jeopardize your journey towards the ultimate goal.

For example, if you are working to keep nervous hunger under control by following a healthy intermittent fasting protocol and during a party you find yourself in front of a tray full of biscuits, do the following things.

- Feel how much you would like to eat those biscuits.

- Recognize that that biscuit could be able to satisfy your current desire for sweets.
- Remember yourself that you are working to achieve the goal of losing 20 pounds by following intermittent fasting protocol and the reward of a new wardrobe.
- Ask yourself if temporary satisfaction given by that biscuit deserves to renounce the progress made and the potential loss of the final award.

Give yourself small rewards for the results achieved

A motivation or reward system will not change your long-term will strength, but you can help you follow the way to success. Since the achievement of a final goal may take a long time, it could be effective to set small rewards for the progress made so that they act as motivation to keep going.

For example, if for a week you have followed your intermittent fasting protocol, you can give yourself a small dose of your favorite dessert over the weekend. Alternatively, you can reward you with something that is not bound to food, like a pedicure or a massage.

Notes your attempts to check your impulses, including both the successful ones and the unsuccessful ones. Don't forget those details that in the future could help you evaluate the situation.

For example, you could write: "Today I ate five cookies during an office party. I had missed lunch and I was quite hungry. I was surrounded by many people and Sara, who had prepared the cookies, repeatedly encouraged me to eat one of them".

Comment on the factors that influenced your decision-making process

In addition to detailing the situation you have resisted or how you have surrendered to the impulse, describe what has passed through your mind in those moments. You may want to include your emotional state, the people you were next to you and the place where you were there.

After describing several episodes in your diary, you can start to re-read them, trying to highlight possible schemes in your behaviors. Here are some questions you should ask yourself.

- Is my decision-making process more effective when I am alone or when I am with other people?
- Are there some people who more than others "trigger" my compulsive behaviors?
- Do my emotions (depression, anger, happiness, etc.) influence my compulsive behavior?
- Is there a particular moment of the day when it is more difficult to keep my impulses under control?

You can decide to create a visual representation of your progress

It may seem to be a strange idea, but there are many women who respond better to a more concrete visual representation of their progress. It will be easier to remain motivated by having something that clearly shows you the many steps taken so far, as well as those still to be done.

For example, if you want to lose 20 pounds, you can insert a coin in a jar whenever you lose 0,5 lbs. Seeing the level of coins grow while losing weight you will have a concrete representation of the progress made.

Find out what is more effective for you

By reading your diary or simply reflecting on your successes and your false steps, you can realize what is more useful for you. You may notice that giving you a weekly reward is really effective. You could then find that being alone is a triggering cause of your compulsive behavior, or that you find yourself in a given place or in the presence of certain people contribute to increasing your food cravings. Customize your approach to increase your willpower based on your specific needs.

Stress can hinder your progress

Whatever health your goal you are trying to reach, stress deriving from working or personal life has the potential to derail your progress. Therefore, it could be necessary to use techniques to reduce your stress. Do not underestimate the influence stress can have in your ability to follow your intermittent fasting protocol.

Sometimes the best way to defeat temptation is to avoid it. If you feel you don't have the willpower needed to resist your compulsive behavior, try to eliminate the opportunity to give up your intermittent fasting protocol. This could mean wanting to avoid those people or those environments that tend to trigger your cravings. This solution may not be valid long-term, but prove to be useful in the beginning of your intermittent fasting protocol or during some particularly difficult moments.

For example, if you tend to eat outside your scheduled eating window, you can decide to empty your home of all sorts of unhealthy food. Remove from your pantry everything that does not suit your new healthy habits, throwing it away.

Use "if-then" affirmations

You can "mentally feel" your reactions at a given situation by inventing some scenarios in advance using the "if-then" structure. Doing this will be particularly useful when you will find yourself in a situation that tempts you.

For example, if you are about to attend a party where biscuits will be available, you can use the following "if - then" statement. "If Sara will offer me a biscuit, then I gently tell her 'no, thanks, but they look delicious' and I'll move to the other side of the room".

<u>Search for medical help</u>

If you have been trying without success to keep your impulses at bay, evaluate the hypothesis to turn to a therapist. They can offer you support and specific tips to change your behaviors.

People suffering from obsessive or compulsive behavior or dependencies can benefit from the help of a therapist specialized in impulse control disorders or cognitive pathologies.Some impulse control disorders and some deficiencies in the willpower can also benefit from a treatment known as "Habit Reversal Therapy" which replaces unwanted habit with another more useful habit.

Chapter 2 - How to Set Your Goals

Whether you have small dreams or high expectations from your intermittent fasting protocol, having goals will allow you to plan your path through this weight loss journey. The achievement of some goals can require a whole life, while others can be conquered from morning to evening. Whatever your goals, broad and generic or specific and practical, in reaching them you will feel satisfied and you will see your self-esteem grow. If the fulfillment of the first necessary steps intimidates you, continue reading and find out how to consolidate the widest desire.

Determine the goals for your life

Ask yourself important questions regarding what you want to get from life. On a physical level, you might want to be back in shape by following an intermittent fasting protocol.

Analyze the areas in which, over time, you would like to make changes or improvements. Start wondering what you want to get in every specific area, and think about what steps you want to take in the next five years.

In the case of the goal "I want to get back in shape", you could establish minor goals as "I want to follow my intermittent fasting protocol" and "I want to fast at least 16 hours a day".

Once you know what you want to get over the next few years, you have to start taking the steps necessary to reach them by writing down the actual goals.

If you want to get back in shape, your first goal may be to eat more fruits and vegetables and run for 3 miles. We will have a chapter dedicated to writing down your goals in the best possible way, for now just know that it is fundamental if you want to lose weight and keep it off.

You have to highlight the reasons why you have decided to set such a goal and reflect on what will happen once you reach it. For example, if referring to a short-term fitness goal you have decided to achieve, it is good to ask yourself if and how your choice will help you reach your main health goal. If necessary, evaluate to change your short-term goal by replacing it with a practice that allows you to effectively advance towards the final destination.

Periodically check your goals

Instead of limiting you to remain anchored on your initial positions, from time to time find time to re-evaluate your minor goals. Are you respecting the temporal deadlines you have set for yourself? Are the steps planned able to lead you to your finish line? Be flexible in changing and adapting your minor goals.

To get back in shape, you may have to follow an intermittent fasting protocol for several weeks. If you start by following a 16/8 intermittent fasting protocol it might be the case for you to take things to a new level by committing yourself to an 18/6 protocol. Have fixed goals but do not be afraid to change your approach to reach them faster.

Make your goals specific

When you set a goal, you have to make sure that you respond to very specific questions: who, what, where and why. For any goal you set, you should reflect on your reasons and ask you how it helps to get you to achieve what you want in life.

To get back in shape (very generic destination), you should create a more specific goal like following an intermittent fasting protocol for a full month. For every goal you set for yourself, you should be as specific and precise as possible. For instance, an example of a well-built goal could be "I am going to lose 10 lbs in one month by following an intermittent fasting protocol".

Measurable goals

In order to be able to track the progress made, your goals should be measurable. "I'm going to follow an intermittent fasting protocol" is a difficult goal to measure and to track compared to "every day I have only an 8 hour window to eat". In practice, you must be able to determine if you have reached your goal or not.

Be realistic when setting up your goals

It is important to evaluate your situation honestly and distinguish realistic goals from unlikely ones. Ask yourself if you have all the tools needed to reach the set goal.

If you don't have the time or interest needed to dedicate many hours to an intermittent fasting protocol every week, this goal is not for you. If this were your case, it will therefore be necessary to choose an alternative path - there are many ways, in fact, to be able to keep yourself in shape without having to follow an intermittent fasting protocol.

At every moment you will have many goals and at different completion stages. You have to decide which are the most important or urgent ones for you. Being committed to achieving too many goals simultaneously will make you feel overwhelmed and will reduce your chances of success. It can be useful to set some main priorities. In this way, when two goals will come into conflict, you will know how to behave. If the choice will fall between completing one or two minority goals or a priority one, you will have no doubt on what to do.

Keep track of the progress made

Writing in a diary allows you to track your progress, both personal and professional and, when you are directed towards a goal, performing an analysis of the steps taken is a great way to keep you motivated. Analyzing your achievements will be a good source of motivation to do better.

Give the right value to the achievement of your goals

Whenever you reach a goal, you should recognize and celebrate your success as it deserves. Reflect on the path that led you to the goal, from the beginning to the end. Evaluate if the goal has satisfied you, evaluate your new skills and knowledge and note if the goal has been reached in full. Once you have reached your goal, just set another one for yourself to keep building on the momentum you have created.

Now that we have seen how to set good goals for a healthier version of you, it is time to analyze how to actually write them down to make sure you have the highest chance of reaching them. After that, we will finally be able to start talking about the most effective intermittent fasting protocols you can follow to lose weight fast.

Nancy Johnson

Chapter 3 - How to Write Down Your Goals for Maximum Results

As we have seen in the previous chapters, a goal is a mental representation of a specific and measurable result that you want to reach through commitment to certain actions. At its base there may be a dream or hope, but unlike dreams a goal is quantifiable. With a well-written goal, you will know what you want to get and how you intend to get it. Writing personal goals can be both incredibly satisfying and widely useful. Some studies have shown that setting goals for your intermittent fasting protocol can help you feel much safer and confident, even when it comes to long-term fasting periods. As the Chinese philosopher Lao Tzu said: "A thousand miles trip starts with a single step". You can start taking the journey that will take you to the desired destination by writing down your personal weight loss goals.

Reflect on what is considered significant

Studies show that when your goals concern something that you consider motivating, you are more likely to reach them. Identify the areas of your life in which you would like to make changes. In this initial phase, it is normal for every area to have rather large borders. Generally, people decide to give themselves goals in terms of self-improvement and physical health. An accurate intermittent fasting protocol can help you move towards these two directions at the same time.

You should start by drafting out your goals on a piece of paper. For example, you may want to make significant changes in areas concerning health and physical well being. Write down this information, specifying what you would like to change.

At this stage you could indicate the goals in vague terms, it is normal. As for health, for example, you could write "improve physical form" or "healthy eating".

Identify your "best self"

Studies suggest that determining which you think is the best possible version of yourself can help you feel more positive and satisfied with your life. No less important, it is a way to understand what are the goals that you really consider significant. Identifying what is the "best yourself as possible" requires two steps. First of all, you have to see yourself in the future, once you reach your goals, and evaluate what are the qualities you need to get to that point.

Imagine a moment in the future when you have become the best possible version of yourself. How will you be? What things will you give more importance to? At this point, it is essential to concentrate on what "yourself" considers important, ignoring the pressures and desires of others.

Imagine the details of this "future you" and think positive. You can think about something that is the "dream of your life", a fundamental stage of your weight loss journey or some other significant result. For example, your best self could be a healthy woman who follows an intermittent fasting protocol with ease. In this case, imagine what you would do. Which intermittent fasting protocol would you follow? How many calories would you eat per day?

Please, put as many details of your best self when writing down your goals. Imagine what qualities your "best self" is using to achieve success. For example, assuming that you are following an intermittent fasting protocol, surely you would know how to meal prep and manage hunger. Those are two skills you just discovered you must develop to improve your health.

Once you have a list of the skills you need to develop, think about which of these qualities you already have. Be honest with yourself, not severe. Then reflect on the qualities you can develop. Imagine ways to be able to develop the habits and skills you need. For example, if you want to follow an intermittent fasting protocol, but you have no knowledge about eating healthy, you can buy a few books about this topic. The beauty of knowledge is that it can be acquired.

Fix priorities for different areas

Once you have filled out a list of areas in which you would like to make changes, you have to put them in order of priority. Trying to improve all aspects of your life at once is likely to end up with you feeling exhausted, running the risk of failing to achieve your goals because they seem impossible.

Divide your goals in three distinct sections:

- General goals
- Second-level goals
- Third-level goals

The first are the most important, because they are the ones who feel more significant to you. Those of the second and third level are relevant, but you do not give them the same value as the general goals. They also tend to be more specific. An example might be helpful. At the general level you might want to "give priority to your health by following an intermittent fasting protocol". At the second level you may want to "be a good friend, keep the house clean, and be a good parent". At the third level you might want to "Learn to knit or become more efficient at work".

Start narrowing the field

When you have established what the areas you would like to change are and what changes you would like to make, you can start determining the specifications of what you would like to achieve. These specifications will be the basis of your goals. By answering some questions you will be able to identify the who, the what, the when, the where and the results you want to achieve.

Studies carried out suggest that formulating a specific goal not only increases the chances of being able to reach it, but it also helps you feel more happy about the changes it requires.

Determine the who

When you formulate a goal, it is important to determine who is responsible for achieving every sub-goal. Since we are talking about personal goals, it is very likely that the responsible is you. Nevertheless, some goals require the cooperation of others, so it is useful to identify who will be responsible for those parts.

For example, "following an intermittent fasting protocol" is a personal goal that probably only involves you. Otherwise, if your goal is "helping my entire family follow an intermittent fasting protocol", it will also be necessary to contemplate the responsibility of other people.

Determine the what

Asking yourself this question helps you to define the goal, the details and results you want to get. For example, "following an intermittent fasting protocol" is a goal too wide to be manageable. It lacks precision. Reflect on the details of what you want to learn to do. "Follow an intermittent fasting protocol and lose 10lbs in 5 weeks" is more specific.

The more details you can add to the what, the clearer the steps you will have to take to achieve your goal.

Determine the when

One of the key factors of correctly formulating your goals is to divide them in different stages. Knowing when you have to reach every specific step can help you stay on the right track, while giving you the clear feeling of being progressing.

Be realistic in setting the different stages you want to reach. "Losing five pounds by following an intermittent fasting protocol" is not something that can occur from one week to another. Reflect on how long it is really necessary to reach every stage of your plan.

Determine the where

In many cases, it may be useful to identify a certain place where you will reach your goal. For example, if what you are pursuing is following an intermittent fasting protocol three times a week, it is good to decide if you intend to cook at home, buy food on the go or have it delivered at your house. It might seem useless to write down so many details, but trust us when we say that they can make or break your ability to achieve your goals.

Determine the how

This step urges you to imagine how you intend to reach every stage of the process to your goal. This way you will define the structure more precisely and you will have a clear idea of the actions you have to do to complete each phase.

Returning to the example of the intermittent fasting protocol, you will need to choose a meal plan, get the ingredients, have the necessary tools and find the time to prepare your meals in the kitchen.

Determine the why

As mentioned above, the chances of being able to achieve your goal increase proportionately to how significant and motivating it feels. Determining the reason behind your goal helps you understand what is the motivation that drives you to achieve a certain goal.

In our example, you may want to follow an intermittent fasting protocol to feel more attractive and be healthy.

It is important to keep the "why" in mind while you do the actions necessary to achieve your goals. Giving you highly specific goals is useful, but you also need to always have a clear motivation that pushes you when things get difficult.

Write your goals in positive terms

Research shows that you are more likely to reach your goals if you express them in positive terms. In other words, write them considering them something towards which you are moving, not something you want to avoid.

For example, if one of your goals is to follow an intermittent fasting protocol, a motivating way to express it would be "eat only from 6pm to midnight".

On the contrary, "not eat from midnight to 6pm" is not very encouraging or motivating. Words become things, so be careful in what words you decide to use.

Make sure your goals are based on performance

Succeeding certainly requires hard work and a strong motivation, but you must also be sure of setting goals that your commitment allows you to reach. The only thing you can control is your actions, not those of others and not the results.

Focus your goals on the actions you can do yourself, instead of specific results. By conceiving success as a performance process, you will be able to feel that you have remained faithful to the commitment taken even on the occasions when the result is not the one you hoped.

Define your strategy

These are the actions and tactics you intend to use to achieve your goals. Break down the strategy in individual concrete tasks as it makes it even easier to put yourself into practice. Furthermore, it helps you monitor progress. Use the answers you gave the previous questions (what, where, when etc.) to be able to determine what your strategy is.

Determine the time frame

Some goals can be achieved more quickly than others. For example, "following an intermittent fasting protocol for a day" is something you can start doing immediately. For other goals, instead, you will have to sustain a much longer effort.

Divide your plan in individual tasks

Once you have determined what is the destination you need to reach, and in what time period you have to do it, you can divide your strategy into smaller and concrete tasks. In practice you can determine the individual actions you have to do to reach that goal. Give yourself a deadline for each one of them to know if you are respecting your plans.

Divide these smaller steps into even smaller tasks

By now, you will probably have noticed the tendency to break down every plan into smaller ones. There is a good reason to do this: research has proven that specific goals are more likely to be achieved, even when they are complex. The reason is that it can be difficult to act in the best way when you do not know what you need to do.

Lists the specific actions you are already taking towards your goal

It is likely that you are already behaving or acting in the correct direction. For example, if you wish to follow an intermittent fasting protocol, you might already be skipping breakfast.

Try to be the most specific possible when you create this list. You could realize you have already completed the tasks or duties without even noticing it. This is a very useful exercise that can give you the feeling of being progressing towards the goal.

Identify what skills you need to learn and develop

With regard to many goals, it is likely that you have not yet developed all the qualities or habits that are needed to reach them. Reflect on what skills and habits you can already count on that are useful to your goal. The exercise of the "best possible version of yourself" can be useful in this case as well.

Make a plan for today

One of the main causes why women fail to achieve their weight loss goals is that they think they have to start to pursue them tomorrow. Think of something you can do today to start putting a part of your plans into practice, it doesn't matter if it is a very small action. The action you have completed today can be of a preparatory type for those you will have to do in the following days. For example, you may notice that you have to collect information before making a certain meal plan for your intermittent fasting protocol. You could browse the web and learn how to cook those foods in the best way. Even a small achievement like this one will provide you with a good dose of the motivation you need to continue.

Identify the obstacles

No one likes to think about the obstacles that can prevent them from succeeding, but it is essential to identify the difficulties you could meet when developing your plan to reach your weight loss goal. This step is useful to make you find ready in case something goes differently from how you planned it. Identify the potential obstacles and actions you will have to take to overcome them.

Fear is one of the main obstacles women face when starting an intermittent fasting protocol. The fear of not being able to get what you want can prevent you from taking productive steps that would allow you to achieve success. The next section of the chapter will teach you to fight your fears using some specific techniques.

Use visualization

Research has shown that visualization may have significant effects on improving your performance. Often, athletes claim that visualizing is the technique at the base of their successes. There are two types of visualization

- Visualization of the result
- Visualization of the process

If you want to have the highest probability of succeeding, you should combine them both.

Visualizing the result means imagining to reach your goal. As for the exercise of the "best self", the visualized image should be the most specific and detailed possible. Use all your senses to create this mental photograph: imagine who is there with you, what smells you perceive, what you hear, how you're dressed, where you are. At this stage of the process, it could be useful to build a vision board.

Visualizing the process means imagining the steps you need to take to be able to achieve your goal. Think of all the actions you have undertaken. The psychologists define it as "prospective memory". This process can help you believe that the tasks you face are feasible. In some cases you will even have the feeling of having already completed them with good results.

Nancy Johnson

Use the power of positive thinking

Some studies have shown that, instead of concentrating on defects and errors, thinking positively can help you adapt better to situations, to learn more easily and change effortlessly. No matter what your goal is: thinking positive is as effective for maximum level athletes as for women that want to lose weight.

Some studies have even demonstrated that positive and negative thinking affect different areas of the brain. Positive thinking stimulates areas of the brain associated with visual processing, imagination, the ability to have detached views, empathy and motivation.

For example, remind yourself that your goals are positive growth experiences instead of something that forces you to avoid certain foods or abandon your habits.

If you have difficulty reaching your goals, ask the support of friends and family.

Recognize the "false hope syndrome"

This is an expression with which psychologists describe a cycle that is probably not foreign to you, if you have written a list of resolutions for the new year before. This cycle is composed of three parts: 1) fix the goal, 2) be surprised to find out how difficult it is to reach that goal 3) give up on the goal.

The same cycle can intervene when you expect to get immediate results (which often happens with resolutions for the new year). Fixing specific temporal strategies and deadlines will help you fight these unrealistic expectations.

The same can happen when the initial enthusiasm, which is born when establishing your goals, vanishes and the only thing that remains is the work you need to do to reach them. Formulating strategies and dividing them in smaller tasks can help you keep the momentum you need. Whenever you carry out an assignment, even the smallest one, you can (and you will have to) celebrate your success.

Consider false steps as opportunities to learn more about yourself

The studies carried out show that women who know how to learn from their mistakes have a more positive vision regarding the possibility of achieving their goals. Optimism is a vital component of success. When you are confident you are more likely to be able to look forward instead of backwards.

Research has also shown that the number of false steps committed by those who reach success is neither lower nor higher than those who surrender. The only difference is given by how women choose to consider their mistakes.

Stop searching for perfection

Often, the search for perfectionism originates from the fear of being vulnerable. In many cases we have the desire to "be perfect" to avoid having to face a defeat or a "failure", but the truth is that perfectionism cannot protect us from these experiences, which are completely natural for human beings. The only result you would get would be to impose standards that are impossible to reach. Several studies have confirmed that there is a very strong link between perfectionism and unhappiness.

Be grateful for who you are right now

Research has shown that there is a considerable bond between the active practice of gratitude and the ability to reach your goals. Keeping a diary of gratitude is one of the simplest and most effective methods to learn to feel grateful in everyday life.

It is not necessary to write a lot. Even one or two sentences regarding a person or experience for which you feel grateful will raise the desired effect.

The idea of keeping such a diary could seem silly or childish, but the truth is that the more you believe its power, the more you can feel grateful and happy. Leave the skeptical thoughts out of the door.

Savor specific moments, even those apparently less relevant. Do not hurry to transcribe them into the diary. Take all the time to enjoy the experience, thoroughly reflecting on its meaning and reasons that make you feel grateful. The studies conducted on the subject have shown that to write every day is less effective than just doing it a few times a week. The reason could be that we tend to lose sensitivity to positive things over time, so make sure you maximize the effects of this method.

If you follow these goal setting strategies we are sure you are going to have an advantage over those women that just decide to start an intermittent fasting protocol without the right mindset.

<u>Chapter 4 - The Basics of Nutrition</u>

Now that we have talked about the right mindset you need to achieve your weight loss goals, it is time to study the basics of nutrition. In fact, by understanding how foods behave once they enter your body, you will discover the best way to eat while following an intermittent fasting protocol. Remember that our goal is to help you lose weight while staying healthy. You should never sacrifice your long term health to lose weight faster. This has never worked out well and never will.

During the evolution of the species, humans have undergone a variation of the alimentary patterns due to a multiplicity of factors. From its origin mankind is omnivorous, able to consume a wide variety of plant and animal materials. It is even noted that omnivorism goes back in time, uniting sandwiches and little men to this diet, differentiating them from other evolutionary lines. In this sense, already from the origins Homo is assimilated to the omnivorism of chimpanzees and bonobo, and relatively distant from the vegetarianism of orangutans.

During different phases of the paleolithic the various hominin species employed hunting, fishing and harvesting as primary sources of food, alternating to the spontaneous plants the animal proteins, and preceding in the evolutionary history the finding of such proteins through saprophagous behaviors (ethology widely spread in H. habilis). It has been proven that the genus Homo has used fire since the time of the predominance of the species Homo erectus that of the fire made documented use, probably also for preparing and cooking food before consuming it. According to Lewis Binford, the feeding of animal carrions has extended to later genera than habilis, involving the so-called Peking Man.

The use of fire has become documented regularly in the species H. sapiens and H. neanderthalensis. It is hypothesized, on a scientific basis, that an evolutionary engine for H. erectus, the first hominid documented to be able to cook food was formed by obtaining, with cooking, more calories from the diet, decrease the hours dedicated to the feeding overcoming the metabolic limitations that in the other primates have not allowed an encephalization and a neuronal development tied to the size of the brain in proportion to the body size. This, combined with an increasing consumption of animal proteins, documented to be ascribed to the Homo-Australopithecus separation, or H. habilis-H. erectus, would have been a powerful evolutionary impulse.

Nutrition is a multifaceted process that depends on the integrity of the functions, such as the introduction of food into the oral cavity, chewing, swallowing, digestion, intestinal transit, absorption and metabolism of nutrients. Human nutrition corresponds to the conscious consumption of food and drink; it is influenced by biological, relational, psychological, sensory or socio-cultural factors. In some periods of life as a newborn or elderly, as well as for some pathologies, an organism may not be able to feed itself autonomously, but it needs assistance. In this case we speak of «assisted nutrition».

When the organism is fed by ways that bypass the natural mode, an «artificial nutrition» is carried out. The medical sciences (human and veterinary) deal with the modalities of administration by artificial routes in case of pathologies involving the apparatuses interested in the introduction of food.

Now that we have done this quick historical introduction, let's take a look at the basic elements of nutrition. We are talking about carbohydrates, fats and proteins.

Chapter 5 - Carbohydrates

Carbohydrates are the most common source of energy in living organisms, and their digestion requires less water than protein or fat. Proteins and fats are structural components needed for organic tissues and cells, and are also a source of energy for most organisms. Carbohydrates in particular are the largest resource for metabolism. When there is no immediate need for monosaccharides they are often converted into more space-friendly forms, such as polysaccharides. In many animals, including humans, this form of storage is glycogen, located in liver and muscle cells. The plants instead use starch as a reserve. Other polysaccharides such as chitin, which contribute to the formation of the exoskeleton of arthropods, instead play a structural function. Polysaccharides are an important class of biological polymers. Their function in living organisms is usually structural or depository. Starch (a glucose polymer) is used as a polysaccharide of deposition in plants, and is found both in the form of amylose and in the branched form of amylopectin. In animals, the structurally similar glucose polymer is the most densely branched glycogen, sometimes called "animal starch". The properties of glycogen allow it to be metabolized more quickly, which adapts to the active lives of moving animals. The most common forms of glycogen are hepatic glycogen and muscle glycogen. Hepatic glycogen is found in the liver, it is the reserve of sugar and energy in animals and lasts 24 hours. Muscle glycogen is the reserve of sugar used directly by muscle cells without passing through blood circulation. Hepatic glycogen, on the other hand, must be introduced into the bloodstream before it reaches the cells and, in particular, muscle tissue. Glucose is relevant in the production of mucin, a protective biofilm of the liver and intestine. The liver must be in a state of excellent health to operate the synthesis of missing glucose from proteins, as is required in low-carb diets. Cellulose is located in cell walls and other organisms, and is believed to be the most abundant organic molecule on Earth. The chitin structure is similar, it has side chains that contain nitrogen, increasing its strength. It is found in the exoskeletons of arthropods and in the cell walls of some fungi.

Role in nutrition

A completely carbohydrate-free diet can lead to ketosis. However, the brain needs glucose to draw energy from: this glucose can be obtained from the milk of nuts, an amino acid present in proteins and also from the glycerol present in triglycerides. Carbohydrates provide 3.75 kcal per gram, proteins 4 kcal per gram, and fats provide 9 kcal per gram. In the case of proteins, however, this information is misleading as only some of the amino acids can be used to derive energy. Similarly, in humans, only some carbohydrates can provide energy, including many monosaccharides and disaccharides. Other types of carbohydrates can also be digested, but only with the help of intestinal bacteria. Ruminants and termites can even digest cellulose, which is not digestible by other organisms. Complex carbohydrates which cannot be assimilated by man, such as cellulose, hemicellulose and pectin, are an important component of dietary fibre. Carbohydrate-rich foods are bread, pasta, legumes, potatoes, bran, rice and cereals. Most of these foods are rich in starch. The FAO (Food and Agriculture Organization) and the WHO (World Health Organization) recommend to ingest 55-75% of the total energy from carbohydrates, but only 10% from simple sugars. The glycemic index and glycemic load are concepts developed to analyze the behavior of food during digestion. These classify carbohydrate-rich foods based on the speed of their effect on blood glucose level. The insulin index is a similar, more recent classification that classifies food by its effect on blood insulin levels, caused by various macronutrients, especially carbohydrates and certain amino acids present in food. The glycemic index is a measure of how quickly carbohydrates of food are absorbed, while the glycemic load is the measure that determines the impact of a given amount of carbohydrates present in a meal.

When you follow an intermittent fasting protocol, during the fasting hours your body is depleted from its carbohydrates reserves and uses fat to fuel your movements and thoughts. This is what allows you to literally melt fat once you reach the last few hours of your fast. It is a powerful concept inspired by nature and it works incredibly well for women of your age.

Chapter 6 - Proteins

In chemistry, proteins (or protids) are biological macromolecules made up of amino acid chains bound together by a peptide bond (a link between the amino group of one amino acid and the carboxylic group of the other amino acid, created through a condensation reaction with loss of a water molecule). Proteins perform a wide range of functions within living organisms, including catalysis of metabolic reactions, synthesis functions such as DNA replication, response to stimuli, and transport of molecules from one place to another. Proteins differ from each other especially in their sequence of amino acids, which is dictated by the nucleotide sequence preserved in the genes and which usually results in protein folding and a specific three-dimensional structure that determines its activity.

By analogy with other biological macromolecules such as polysaccharides and nucleic acids, proteins form an essential part of living organisms and participate in virtually every process that takes place within cells. Many are part of the category of enzymes, whose function is to catalyze biochemical reactions vital to the metabolism of organisms. Proteins also have structural or mechanical functions, such as actin and myosin in the muscles and proteins that make up the cytoskeleton, which form a structure that allows the cell to be maintained. Others are essential for inter- and intracellular signal transmission, immune response, cell adhesion and cell cycle. Proteins are also necessary elements in animal nutrition, since they cannot synthesize all the amino acids they need and must obtain the essential ones through food. Thanks to the digestion process, the animals break down the proteins ingested in the individual amino acids, which are then used in the metabolism.

Once synthesized in the organism, proteins exist only for a certain period of time and then are degraded and recycled through cellular mechanisms for the protein turnover process. The duration of a protein is measured in terms of half-life and can be very varied. Some may exist for only a few minutes, others up to a few years. However, the average lifespan in mammalian cells is between 1 and 2 days. Abnormal and misfolded proteins can cause instability if they are not degraded more quickly.

Proteins can be purified from other cellular components using a variety of techniques such as ultracentrifugation, precipitation, electrophoresis and chromatography. The advent of genetic engineering has made possible a number of methods to facilitate such purification. Commonly used methods to study protein structure and function include immunohistochemistry, site-specific mutagenesis, X-ray crystallography, nuclear magnetic resonance imaging. The proteins differ mainly for the sequence of the amino acids that compose them, which in turn depends on the nucleotide sequence of the genes that express the synthesis within the cell.

A linear chain of amino acid residues is called "polypeptide" (a chain of several amino acids bound by peptide bonds). A protein generally consists of one or more long polypeptides that may be coordinated with non-peptide groups, called prosthetic groups or cofactors. Short polypeptides, containing less than about 20-30 amino acids, are rarely considered proteins and are commonly called peptides or sometimes oligopeptides. The sequence of amino acids in a protein is defined by the sequence present in a gene, which is encoded in the genetic code. In general, the genetic code specifies 20 standard amino acids. However, in some organisms the code may include selenocysteine (SEC), and in some archaea, pyrrolysine, and finally a 23rd amino acid, N-formylmethionine, a methionine derivative, which initiates protein synthesis of certain bacteria.

Shortly after or even during protein synthesis, protein residues are often chemically modified by post-translational modification, which if present alters physical and chemical properties, bending, stability, activity and ultimately, the function of the protein. Proteins can also work together to achieve a particular function and often associate in stable multiprotein complexes.

Proteins that contain the same type and number of amino acids may differ from the order in which they are located in the structure of the molecule. This aspect is very important because a minimal variation in the sequence of amino acids of a protein (that is in the order in which the various types of amino acids follow each other) can lead to variations in the three-dimensional structure of the macromolecule which can make the protein non-functional. A well-known example is the case of the human hemoglobin beta chain, which in its normal sequence carries a trait formed by the following proteins: valine-histidine-leucine-threonine-proline-glutamic acid-lysine.

Proteins and nutrition

The biological value of a protein identifies its ability to meet the metabolic needs of the body for total amino acids and essential amino acids.

The protein quality varies according to the digestibility of the protein (% digested amount and amount of amino acids absorbed in the gastrointestinal tract) and its composition in essential amino acids.

Foods of animal origin (meat, cold cuts, fish, eggs, milk and dairy products) have high biological quality proteins because they contain all the essential amino acids in adequate quantities and are easy to digest. For this reason they are also called noble proteins or high biological value .

Cereals (bread, pasta, rice, spelt, etc.) and legumes (chickpeas, peas, soya, beans, etc.), being of vegetable origin, contain proteins with reduced biological value and that is of inadequate quality. In fact, on the one hand they are not digestible, on the other they do not contain, or contain in insufficient quantity, some essential amino acids.

To ensure protein completeness, even by consuming foods of vegetable origin, it is essential to combine cereals and legumes by consuming traditional Mediterranean dishes. We are talking about pasta and beans, legume soups with spelt/barley, rice and peas, etc. These foods, consumed together, provide a good quantity and quality of amino acids similar (but not equal) to food of animal origin.

Protein daily requirement

The daily protein requirement of a subject depends on several factors, such as age, sex, body weight, physiological-nutritional status and physical activity.

It should be remembered that the body does not stock protein, so it is important to meet the daily protein requirement ensuring the correct amount of essential amino acids.

Based on the LARN requirements (Reference Nutrient Intake Levels - IV revision 2014) and the quality of the proteins introduced by the American population, it has been calculated, on average, how much protein should be taken by age, sex, and weight. For women over 50 years of age, it is recommended one gram of protein for every pound of body weight. So, if you are 120 lbs, you should get at least 60 grams of proteins per day.

Correct intake of protein

To fully exploit all the potential of proteins, it is necessary to make an optimal use so that they are not "dispersed" because they are used as energy. The energy needed for the human body must come mainly from carbohydrates and fats, so that only a part of the protein is used as energy. Protein foods, in particular of animal origin, must be consumed at main meals, e.g.:

The so-called dissociated diets, which provide only proteins or only carbohydrates, not only do not work, but, without introducing on every meal carbohydrates and fats, proteins are consumed thus establishing a protein-energy malnutrition. Obviously the energy introduced must respect the energy balance. You have to introduce as much as you consume, otherwise the macronutrients in excess (proteins or fats or carbohydrates) are stored in your belly. Another important factor is low-calorie and high-protein diets. The diet of protein alone must be prescribed by the nutritionist doctor who limits its consumption over time and in the quality of nutrients. High-protein diets, or DIY diets can make you quickly lose a few extra pounds, but they also often consume lean-mass proteins (muscles, etc.) and thereby reduce the metabolic capacity of the body so that when you go back to eating normally, you take back that pounds.

Chapter 7 - Fats

Lipids are an important energy reserve for animals and plants, as they are able to release a large amount of calories per unit mass. The caloric value of one gram of lipids is about twice as high as sugar and protein, about 9.46 kcal/g versus 4.15 kcal/g. That's why they are the ideal energy substrate for cells. In a healthy woman of 120lbs, there are about 25lbs of fat. During physical activity lipids are used together with carbohydrates, providing the same amount of energy for medium-low level activities. If physical activity lasts for at least an hour you encounter a depletion of carbohydrate stocks (glycogen) and a corresponding increase in the use of lipids. In addition, food lipids provide essential fatty acids (that is, not synthesized by the body), such as linoleic acids (from which arachidonic acid derives) and linolenic.

In a balanced and healthy diet it is important to limit the consumption of saturated and hydrogenated fats, as they entail an increased cardiovascular risk and prefer, instead, unsaturated fats such as those represented by extra virgin olive oil and those present in fish or oil seeds.

The recommended daily intake varies from 25 % to 35 % of total daily calories. Olive oil contains monounsaturated fats and a whole series of other nutrients such as polyphenols with antioxidant function, vitamin E and anticancer compounds: olive oil is the main food of the Mediterranean diet and must never be missed on your dishes.

Blue fish (salmon, tuna, mackerel, sardines) contains polyunsaturated fats of the omega 3 series. These fats are called essential, because the human body is not able to synthesize them and must be introduced from the outside with food. In recent years, numerous studies have highlighted the vital importance of these lipids, as they have many beneficial effects on our health and even in the prevention of many diseases (premature aging, heart attacks, depression, Alzheimer's, senile dementia, etc.).

Oilseeds are valuable and very useful foods to eat as they contain fat-soluble vitamins, minerals such as magnesium and polyunsaturated essential fats similar to those contained in fish. Almonds, walnuts, hazelnuts, linseed, pumpkin seeds, sunflower seeds, sesame seeds, pistachios, cashews, etc. can be inserted in the daily diet by adding them, for example, to salads or consumed at breakfast or in the snack.

Hydrogenated and trans fats, contained for example in vegetable margarine and in some oils such as rapeseed oil, are to be avoided. In fact, they are harmful to cell membranes and increase LDL cholesterol, blocking even some mitochondrial breathing processes. Unfortunately, these fats are very present in baked and packaged products, so it is important to always read the labels and check their absence.

Nancy Johnson

Chapter 8 - Vitamins

Vitamins, essential organic compounds in many vital processes, are not synthesized by the body, so it is necessary to integrate them through nutrition. The amounts needed are very small (some milligrams or micrograms per day) and for this reason they are considered micronutrients, in contrast to macronutrients (carbohydrates, fats and proteins) that should be taken in much larger amounts, or tens or hundreds of grams a day. Vitamins are divided into fat-soluble and water-soluble vitamins, based on their solubility in fat and water.

Fat-soluble vitamins

Vitamin A refers to a series of compounds that in nature are found in different forms: retinol and retinal acid. Plant precursors of vitamin A are carotenoids, mainly beta-carotene. This vitamin is essential for cell differentiation, foetal development, immune system, skin and vision. Its deficiency causes mainly night blindness, dryness of the cornea and opacization and corneal ulcerations, while its excess induces fetal malformations, liver damage and, in the case of ingestions of very high quantities, cerebral edema and coma. The recommended daily dose corresponds to 6-700 µg. It is contained in milk, butter, cheese, eggs and, in general, in foods containing animal fats. Carotenoids and beta-carotene are present in colored vegetables.

Vitamin D exists in two forms: cholecalciferol, or vitamin D3, and ergocalciferol, or vitamin D2. Cholecalciferol is mainly synthesized by the body and is formed in the skin by the effect of sunlight; ergocalciferol is taken with food. Both of these forms require activation by the kidney and liver that transform them into 25-hydroxy-vitamin D. In this form, vitamin D promotes intestinal calcium absorption, renal phosphorus elimination and the release of calcium from the bone. Vitamin D deficiency causes osteomalacia, a condition in which the mineral component of the bone is reduced with consequent fractures caused by even minimal trauma. Psychological symptoms such as depression and neurological symptoms such as neuromyopathy may be associated. Under normal renal function conditions, the dosage of 25-hydroxy-vitamin D is a good indicator of its state. Vitamin D deficiencies may be due to reduced dietary intake, poor exposure to sunlight, malabsorption (intestinal diseases), kidney and liver failure. The best food sources are milk and its derivatives. The daily intake recommended by Larns (recommended nutrient levels) is dependent on solar exposure. During pregnancy and lactation 10 µg per day are recommended.

Vitamin E includes 8 compounds, 4 belonging to the class of tocopherols and 4 to that of tocotrienols. It is mainly found in vegetable oils, fruits and oilseeds and the daily recommended amount depends on the amount of unsaturated fat intake. The main biological activity of vitamin E is the antioxidant one, which mainly occurs in lipid environments, such as cell membranes and lipoproteins, where there is a need to defend from oxidation the double bonds of unsaturated fatty acids. Deficiency symptoms are extremely rare and manifest with peripheral neuropathy, altered coordination of movements, myopathy and retinopathy. The determination of plasma levels of vitamin E is a good indicator of the adequacy of its intake.

Vitamin K includes a series of compounds belonging to two families: phylloquinone, substances present in the plant kingdom, and menaquinones, produced in the intestine by the bacterial flora. Vitamin K is essential for the synthesis of certain coagulation factors by the liver. Recently, it has been shown its role also in the metabolism of the bone. Vitamin K deficiency leads to a blood clotting deficit with reduced prothrombin time. Women over 50 are considered adequate contributions between 60 and 80 µg per day. Vitamin K is contained in vegetables, especially in broad-leaved green plants and in the liver.

Water-soluble vitamins

Thiamine, in the form of thiamine pyrophosphate, plays a key role in the metabolism of carbohydrates and branched-chain amino acids. In its absence, glucose is only partially metabolized, resulting in the formation of excess lactic acid. Deficiency of this vitamin causes heart failure, peripheral neuropathy, coma and intellectual and memory impairments. Minor deficits can result in weakness, reduced appetite, and psychological changes. The requirement is about 1-1.2 milligrams per day (0.5 mg per 1000 kcal introduced). In conditions where metabolic activity increases, such as exercise, pregnancy, and certain diseases, the body needs more vitamin B1. Its dosage in the blood is technically complex and is not performed routinely. It is found in food of animal origin (meat, milk and dairy products, eggs), legumes, whole grains and yeast.

Also called riboflavin, vitamin B2 is a substance that becomes part of enzymes involved in energy metabolism. Its deficiency manifests with lesions in the corners of the lips, glossitis and seborrheic dermatitis. The requirement is 1.3-1.6 mg per day. It is present in numerous foods, such as meat, dairy products, eggs, legumes, whole grains, yeast, vegetables.

Niacin can be synthesized by the body from a protein amino acid, tryptophan. Niacin deficiency gives rise to pellagra: the name given to this vitamin, PP or Pellagra Preventing, is to indicate its effectiveness in preventing this disease, which initially manifests itself with skin lesions, then with intestinal disorders (diarrhea) and finally dementia. The recommended daily intake is 14-18 mg. It is mainly found in meats, dairy products, eggs, legumes, whole grains and yeast.

Pyridoxine is a vitamin mainly involved in amino acid metabolism. Its deficiency causes seborrheic dermatitis and microcytic anemia due to reduced synthesis of hemoglobin. The recommended intake is 1.1-1.5 mg per day. It is mainly found in meat, dairy products, eggs, legumes, whole grains and yeast.

Vitamin B12 is involved in many processes, including the synthesis of nucleic acids and the metabolism of amino acids. To be absorbed at the intestinal level, it must bind with the intrinsic factor, a substance produced by the stomach that has the task to protect it in its path from the stomach bottom to the blood flow. Some gastric diseases, as well as surgical removal of the stomach, cause vitamin B12 deficiency. This deficiency manifests with an anemia characterized by increased red blood cell size, increased plasma levels of homocysteine, atrophy of the lingual papillae, glossitis, neurological damage with disorders of coordination and motor skills, even irreversible. Vitamin B12 can be easily measured in the blood. The recommended daily intake is 2 µg. It is made exclusively from animal sources, so vegan diets easily expose its deficiency.

Folates are a group of substances characterized by a chemical structure similar to that of folic acid; some of their functions are similar to those of vitamin B12. They also fall into enzymatic complexes involved in the metabolism of nucleic acids and amino acids. Deficiency occurs with megaloblastic anemia and increased plasma levels of homocysteine. The dose of folate in plasma is a commonly performed survey and is a good indicator of the state of this vitamin. The recommended daily quantity is 200 µg (400 µg in pregnancy). Good sources of folate are fresh vegetables.

Vitamin C consists of ascorbic acids and hydrocarbons. Its function is complex, intervening in redox reactions, in the synthesis of collagen (the most important structural protein of our organism), in the antioxidant activity in the aqueous phase, in the regeneration of vitamin E and glutathione (antioxidant endogenous substance) oxidized. Vitamin C deficiency causes scurvy, a disease characterized by vascular fragility with gingival bleeding, joint bleeding, petechiae (skin spots due to the breaking of small vessels), susceptibility to infection, weakness and apathy. Vitamin C can be measured in plasma, as an index of recent intakes, and in leukocytes, as an index of reserves. It is recommended to take 60 mg per day. It is found mainly in fresh vegetables and large quantities are contained in citrus fruits and kiwis.

Biotin is a vitamin involved in energy metabolism, as a component of mitochondrial enzymes. Its deficiency, rarely observable, manifests with dermatitis, conjunctivitis and alopecia. It is believed that the necessary doses are between 30 and 100 µg per day. Biotin is made from many animal and plant foods and is also synthesized from intestinal bacterial flora.

Chapter 9 - The Secret Formula to Lose Weight

We assume that to lose weight there are no secrets, or miracle diets, or miracle professionals, but there are methods that can be applied differently according to lifestyle and your energy needs. It is also important that constancy and time are our friends. Beyond the type of diet that can be more or less effective, you have to have patience in losing weight. You will see that by losing just 4 lbs you will feel much more deflated and you will be stimulated to continue in the nutritional path.

Caloric Deficit

To understand the meaning of calorie deficit we must first understand the difference between caloric needs and caloric income. The caloric requirement is the energy that our body needs to support all our physiological functions, basal metabolism, physical activities and daily activities.

Theoretically, if we consume as many calories as our caloric requirements, we remain constant with weight. At a time when our caloric intake is greater than our energy needs, we increase in weight. On the contrary, if we consume less calories than our energy needs we will create a calorie deficit and therefore lose weight.

All this, however, is not a perfect mathematical equation, as there are mechanisms that tend to adapt the metabolism when we eat more or eat less. This means that when we take a calorie surplus, a part of it is turned into heat, while when we create a calorie deficit not all the deficit will be turned into weight loss, but the metabolism will adapt to the daily calorie restriction. These are the reasons why we don't get fat or lose weight forever. In fact, our organism has mechanisms of adaptation so that it does not succumb to hunger in the short and medium term. Of course, a calorie deficit that lasts for life as well as a calorie excess that lasts for life will lead on the one hand to malnutrition and then to death, on the other to metabolic diseases and over time to death for cardiovascular diseases.

How to calculate your calorie deficit

To calculate your calorie deficit and therefore know how many calories you have to eat to lose weight, you have to know your starting point, that is, you have to know your current daily calorie intake. To do this you must write down everything you eat daily for at least five days, in which at least one of these must be a holiday day where you will eat more than normal. To know the calories consumed daily, you can make use of some well-made and easy to use applications. The most used are Myfitnesspal and Yazio. First, before you start your food diary, weigh yourself and then write down everything you bring to your mouth. Once you know the calories you consume in these five days you'll have to average them. The value obtained is most likely your daily calorie intake.

Many women when they write down everything they eat tend to self-regulate. The consequence of self-regulation is that they will tend to eat less than they previously ate because of the awareness they acquire about their diet. So if you weigh yourself after five days of a food diary, and you've had a slight weight loss, add an extra 5% to your average. This percentage gap is probably what made you lose weight.

How to go in calorie deficit

Once you get the value with your application, you have to figure out how to go into a calorie deficit. The method consists in eliminating enough calories to allow weight loss to happen. Suppose you have a daily caloric intake of 2200kcal. Theoretically to have a weight loss of 500 gr per week you will have to eliminate 500 kcal per day from your current calorie income. Therefore, if you want to lose 500 gr per week you will have to eat 1700kcal per day. Our experience tells us that this calorie cut is relatively sustainable.

In order for the diet to be sustainable and not to allow the metabolism to adapt to the calorie deficit, it must not always be the same, but must change day by day. This means that in a week you will have to eat about 12000 kcal. These calories you can distribute as you want, the important thing is that at the end of the week you will have eaten 12000 kcal. For example, from Monday to Saturday you can eat 1500 kcal and on Sunday 3000 kcal. Of course don't weigh yourself the next Monday as you might have a little more water retention.

Wait for next Wednesday. Alternatively you could also do a day of 1500 kcal and a day of 1900 kcal. Basically you can manage the diet however you want, the important thing is that it is from 12 thousand kcal weekly.

This method helps you to follow a more conscious and flexible and less rigid intermittent fasting protocol.

How to build the diet based on the caloric deficit obtained

To build your diet based on the calorie deficit you calculated, with the same application you used to make your food diary, you can build your diet based on your work needs, your schedule and your food tastes. From these choices, however, you will have to have some basic rules, otherwise you will tend to always eat the same foods or the one you prefer. Remember that a diet should also be a healthy food lifestyle that helps you change your wrong habits. Therefore try to eat legumes at least twice a week in the absence of an irritable colon, at least twice a week eggs and prefer white meats to red meats and sausages.

If you can't lose weight then you'll probably have to investigate the reasons for your difficulty. A simple method to stimulate your metabolism is to create a calorie deficit for 4 days a week, and then 3 days of normal calorie diet that in the example case would be 4 days of 1700 kcal and 3 days of 2200kcal.

This method will have to be followed for at least 2 months. Of course, in this way, the weight loss will be slower, but necessary to see an improvement in the efficiency of the metabolism. To improve the efficiency of your metabolism you can keep training as well.

There are also some cases in which you still can not lose weight, despite the metabolic stimulus. In this case it is necessary an impedance to identify the metabolic cell mass and in more serious cases it is necessary to do an indirect colorimetry to understand the proper functioning of the metabolism or alternatively hematologic analysis to identify if there are hormonal problems.

<u>Conclusion</u>

We would like to thank you for making it to the end of this intermittent fasting guide. We have done our best to ensure that every information contained is useful and helps you in your journey towards a healthier you.

We know how frustrating it could be to start an intermittent fasting protocol and feeling discouraged by the fact that results do not appear immediately. As we repeated throughout this entire guide, the goal of intermittent fasting is to create a healthy lifestyle that can support you over the years, not just give you a rapid weight loss that is unsustainable over the long run.

By following the intermittent fasting protocols and strategies shared in this book, you will certainly burn fat, lose weight and feel much better. However, as we do not know you in person, our final recommendation can only be the following one.

Before starting an intermittent fasting protocol talk to your doctor and find out whether intermittent fasting could be a good idea for you or not. Remember, never sacrifice your health to fit into that new skirt you just got.

Be healthy and your weight will adapt.

To your success!

Nancy Johnson

Weight Loss for Beginners

Intermittent Fasting and OMAD Diet

Discover how to Lose Weight, Burn Fat and Detoxify Your Body with the Incredible 16/8 Fasting Method - Weight Loss Strategies to Live Longer Included!

By

Nancy Johnson

render any resulting actions solely under their purview. There are no scenarios in which the publisher or the original author of this work can be in any fashion deemed liable for any hardship or damages that may befall them after undertaking information described herein.

Additionally, the information in the following pages is intended only for informational purposes and should thus be thought of as universal. As befitting its nature, it is presented without assurance regarding its prolonged validity or interim quality. Trademarks that are mentioned are done without written consent and can in no way be considered an endorsement from the trademark holder.

Weight Loss for Beginners

Table of Contents

Introduction

Most women over 50 feel as if they have lost their ability to be attractive, healthy and feel good in their own bodies. This is due to the fact that in today's world, we are spending more and more time at home and we have significantly reduced our need for food. However, even if we do not need as many calories as we did in the past, most of us are still eating as if they were running a marathon a day.

Therefore, it should not come as a surprise that most women over 50 are out of shape, overweight and unhealthy. Thanks to researches and scientific studies conducted by incredible nutritionists, it is now possible to overcome the negative effect of a sedentary life. In fact, intermittent fasting seems like the perfect solution for all those women that want to burn fat, lose weight and gain a healthy and new lifestyle.

The need of all these women is what inspired the writing of this book. In fact, in the next chapters you are not going to find complicated explanations of scientific topics that, even if interesting, do not give you a clear direction on what you can do to start feeling better. On the contrary, while writing this book, a great effort was made to make sure that each concept is followed by a subsequent strategy that can be implemented in a healthy intermittent fasting protocol.

By reading this book you will get all the information and practical steps you need to follow to start intermittent fasting in just a few days. We advise you to talk to your doctor before changing your diet as intermittent fasting is not suitable if you have certain healthy conditions.

Please, be aware that the goal of this book is to give you accurate information on intermittent fasting, but it does not take the place of a professional opinion. We hope that you can find motivational and informative insights that help you make a change for the better.

To your success!

Nancy Johnson

<u>Chapter 1 - An Introduction to Fasting</u>

Before beginning our discussion about intermittent fasting, it is important to have a good understanding of what fasting actually is in a more general sense. In the next few pages we are going to lay out the basics for the rest of the book, so pay close to attention.

Although cases of prolonged fasting due to lack of food are extremely rare in our society, voluntary food deprivation is often undertaken for political, social or religious reasons. Since humans can survive absolute fasting for about 24-30 days, the body's physiological response to this deprivation can be divided into 4 phases, respectively called the post-absorption period, short fasting, medium fasting and prolonged fasting. Let's take a look at them one by one to understand them better.

Post-absorption period
It occurs a few hours after the last food intake, as soon as the foods introduced in the last meal have been completely

absorbed by the intestine. On average it lasts three or four hours, followed, under normal conditions, by an ingestion of food that breaks the temporary state of fasting.

In the post-absorption period there is a progressive accentuation of hepatic glycogenolysis ("breakdown" of glycogen into the individual glucose units that make it up), which is necessary to cope with the glycemic drop and supply extrahepatic tissues with glucose.

Short-term fasting

In the first 24 hours of food deprivation, metabolism is supported by the oxidation of triglycerides and glucose deposited in the liver in the form of glycogen. Over time, given the modest amount of hepatic glycogen stores, most of the tissues (muscle, heart, kidney, etc.) adapt to use mainly fatty acids, saving glucose. The latter will be destined above all to the brain and anaerobic tissues such as red blood cells which, in order to "survive", absolutely need glucose. In fact, they cannot use fatty acids for energy purposes. Under similar conditions, the cerebral demands for glucose amount to 4 g/hour, while those of the anaerobic tissues amount to 1.5 g/hour. Since the liver cannot obtain more than 3g of glucose per hour from glycogenolysis, it is forced to activate an "emergency" metabolic pathway, called gluconeogenesis. This process consists in the production of glucose starting from amino acids.

Fasting of medium duration

If food deprivation lasts beyond 24 hours, the action described in the adaptation phase continues with a progressive accentuation of gluconeogenesis. The amino acids necessary to satisfy this process derive from the breakdown of muscle proteins. Since there are no protein deposits in the body to be used for energy purposes, the body, in order to survive the fast, is forced to "cannibalize" its muscles. This process is accompanied by an inevitable reduction in muscle mass, with the consequent appearance of weakness and apathy.

In the early stages, gluconeogenesis is capable of producing over 100g of glucose per day, but soon enough the efficiency of this process decreases to around 75 g/day. Unlike what happens during the first phase, this quantity is no longer sufficient to ensure an adequate supply of glucose to the brain. Therefore, this organ is forced to increasingly resort to ketone bodies, three water-soluble molecules deriving from the oxidation of fats in conditions of glucose deficiency. The overproduction of ketone bodies (a process called ketosis), while prolonging the survival of the organism by a few days, causes an important increase in blood acidity.

During fasting periods of medium duration, which extends up to the twenty-fourth day of food deprivation, the recourse of other tissues to lipid oxidation increases more and more, with a general view of maximum saving of blood glucose.

Prolonged fasting and death

This phase begins when the fast lasts beyond the 24th day. The body has now exploited all the protein resources, including plasma proteins. The mix of ketosis, the lowering of the immune defenses, the dehydration and the reduced respiratory efficiency (given by the catabolism of the proteins of the diaphragm and intercostal muscles) condemns the individual to an unfortunate fate.

So should you be afraid of fasting? That's a reasonable question and if you bought this book is because you are interested in seeing what it can do to help you lose weight. Let's be clear from the start: no, fasting is a great solution to burn fat and get healthier. However, there are some important things to point out to avoid making bad mistakes that can result in health damages.

Many people resort to fasting driven by fashions, advertising or food and health beliefs that are at least questionable. Voluntary abstinence from food intake is understood, in these cases, as a moment of physical purification, aimed at eliminating toxins accumulated due to an incorrect diet.

To analyze this fact, after having broadly described the biochemical aspects, we can start from two assumptions. The first, irrefutable, is that we have plenty of food available, a high-calorie food that is often the basis of obesity; in short, we eat too much and the consequences are there for everyone to see. In fact, overeating and a sedentary lifestyle are among the very first causes of death in industrialized countries, including the US. The second point is that a moderately low-calorie diet, summarized in the Japanese saying "hara hachi bu" (get up from the table with an 80% full stomach), is one of the best strategies for living longer and healthier.

While many people should cut down on their food intake, there is no need to resort to extreme solutions such as prohibitive diets or fasting. Instead, it is enough, as our grandparents used to say, to get up from the table when you are still a little hungry and keep in mind that a little exercise never hurts.

Fasting, similar to physical activity, is a stress for the body. The difference is that, while sport leads to an improvement in organic abilities, fasting moves in the opposite direction. The lack and prolonged intake of nutrients reduces muscle mass and basal metabolism (up to 40% in extreme cases). Furthermore, the mind becomes cloudy and a global state of debilitation arises, characterized by a decrease in muscle strength and ability to concentrate. All this has nothing therapeutic or detoxifying.

Partial or attenuated fasting, on the other hand, could have positive implications, as long as it is applied rationally. After a Christmas dinner, for example, it is useful to follow a low-calorie diet rich in liquids and vegetables for two or three days. The important thing is to associate these foods with a certain amount of proteins, perhaps obtained from lean fish (which is usually easy to digest), and fats, for example by consuming a handful of dried fruit. In this way you avoid "cannibalizing your muscles" and depressing your metabolism excessively and then paying the consequences. This last point must also be clear to those who resort to fasting in extremis to lose weight before summer. In fact, a few pounds can be lost but the amount of energy associated with each unit of weight lost is very low. In other words, weight loss is mainly linked to increased diuresis and muscle catabolism induced by prolonged fasting.

As you might have noticed, even if this book is about intermittent fasting for weight loss, we are not advocating the use of fasting without pointing out the importance of doing things the proper way. In fact, the main reason we decided to write this book is to share the right information that can actually make a difference when starting out with intermittent fasting. Your health is extremely important and we would never advise you to do extreme things just to lose a few pounds.

Now that we are done with this disclaimer, we can finally focus on how you can use intermittent fasting to start losing fat.

Chapter 2 - HIIT: A Particular Type of Training

Let's start our discussion on how to follow a healthy intermittent fasting protocol by taking a look at the type of training that we recommend the most.

There is a specific type of training that we recommend to all those women that are looking to combine strength and cardio into one simple routine. We are talking about HIIT and the next few pages are going to tell you everything there is to know about it.

High Intensity Interval Training consists of alternating short and very intense efforts, therefore with a large anaerobic component, with less intense recovery periods until muscle and / or metabolic exhaustion is reached.

Duration and intensity of the peaks are inversely proportional, since the effort should be maximal or sub-maximal. Although there is no precise and advisable total duration, HIIT workouts generally last less than 30 minutes, with times that can vary according to your personal level of training.

HIIT training sessions generally consist of the following phases.

- General and specific warm up

- Repetition or series of high intensity (HIT) exercises, separated by low or medium intensity executions as active recovery

- Cool down and some exercises for flexibility and mobility.

HIT should be performed at maximum intensity, while active recovery should not have an intensity greater than 50%. The number of sets/reps and the duration of each depend on the type of exercise, but can be as little as 3 reps of 20 seconds each. The specific exercises performed during times of high intensity can vary even within the same workout. Most of the research on HIIT has been done using a cycling ergometer (stationary bike), but you can use whatever cardio equipment you have at your disposal.

There is no specific formula of HIIT. Depending on your cardiovascular and muscular level, the recovery intensity can be medium or very slow; what matters are the high intensity peaks. A common formula is a 2: 1 ratio of high intensity to active recovery, such as 30–40" of fast running alternating with 15-20" of jogging or walking, repeated "X" times or until exhaustion.

The entire HIIT session can last from 4 to 30 minutes, which means it is considered an excellent way to maximize your training in the event of time constraints. The use of a watch or timer is highly recommended to respect exercise, recovery times and to estimate beats per minute (bpm) - alternatively, a heart rate monitor is very useful.

Intensity VS Volume

Intensity and volume are two parameters which, together with density, constitute the workload. In fact, the formula to calculate the total load is this:

intensity + volume + density = TOT load

HIIT is based, as mentioned above, on HIT (high intensity training), to which it associates IT (interval training) to be able to increase its total volume.

However, it must be said that "high intensity" is a relative concept, in the sense that it can be applied to efforts of a different nature, and which use equally different metabolisms. It is in fact common to speak of high volume training and low intensity for all undemanding aerobic endurance activities: light running for an hour, cycling for 2-3 hours, brisk walking for 90 seconds and everything in between.

In this case the intensity is objectively low; what happens though, if we report the same concept on protocols that basically stimulate the metabolisms of anaerobic intensities?

In strength training, the concept does not fundamentally change; yet the metabolisms recruited are mainly anaerobic, alactacid and lactacid. Why do we make this clarification? To distinguish the various training strategies, which obviously have different purposes.

Thinking about the training of a bodybuilder, knowing that muscle mass is sought by orienting programming in different directions, we could deduce phases with different characteristics:

- Concentric "pure" strength development: for example, with a short and rapid table, in multi-frequency in the micro cycle, based on a few exercises of 5 sets x 5 rep at 90% of 1RM, low TUT (times of muscle tension), in which the recovery is almost full

- Search for hypertrophy due to depletion of energy supplies, high production of lactic acid emphasis on isometry and eccentric phases of contraction: with long sessions of 10-12 rep at 75% of the 1RM x 4 sets, with shorter, higher recovery time, many more exercises, almost always in single frequency in the micro cycle.

This last method, which objectively prolongs the training up to 75-90', against the 30-40' of the previous one, in the context of training for muscle strengthening, can be considered a high volume and lower intensity system - also it has nothing to do with the long walks we talked about above.

HIIT is designed to increase training efficiency, both in terms of physical conditioning (muscle and metabolic), and from the point of view of infra and post exercise caloric consumption - Excess Postexercise Oxygen Consumption (EPOC) or "afterburn" or debt of post exercise oxygen.

By training in HIIT it is possible to gain a better physical condition and a higher athletic ability. In this case, High Intensity Interval Training determines an improvement in glucose metabolism (sensitivity to glucose and insulin).

HIIT vs Low Intensity High Volume Training (LIHVT)

Compared to aerobic "Low Intensity High Volume Training" (LIHVT), HIIT "may" not be as effective for:

- Treatment of hyperlipidemias, in which low intensity and prolonged training seems to act more by reducing triglyceridemia and improving cholesterolemia

- Treatment of severe obesity and uncomfortable conditions or pathologies, such as severe heart disease, broncho pneumopathies (e.g. COPD) etc.
- Muscle and bone mass restoration in subjects suffering from sarcopenia, osteopenia and osteoporosis.

However, research has shown that HIIT regimens can induce - for the same caloric intake compared to LIHVT - significant reductions in body fat mass.

Other insights, however, have highlighted that HIIT requires an extremely high level of personal motivation by questioning whether the general population can safely or practically tolerate the extreme nature of the method. This is particularly true for those that have never embraced a healthy lifestyle before.

Benefits

We now list the health effects of High Intensity Interval Training.

Cardiovascular benefits of HIIT

A 2015 systematic review and meta-analysis of randomized trials found that HIIT training and LIHVT training both lead to significant improvement in cardiovascular fitness in healthy adults aged 18 to 45. However, greater improvements in VO2 max were observed in those participating in the HIIT exercise regimen.

Another analysis also found that HIIT regimens of 30 days or longer effectively improve cardiovascular fitness in teens and lead to moderate improvements in body composition.

Additionally, a separate systematic review and meta-analysis of seven small randomized trials found that HIIT (defined as four four-minute intervals at 85-95% of maximum heart rate with three-minute intervals at 60-70% of FcMax) was more effective than continuous moderate-intensity training at improving blood vessel function and blood vessel health markers.

HIIT and cardiovascular disease

A 2015 meta-analysis comparing HIIT with moderate intensity continuous training (MICT) in individuals with coronary artery disease found that HIIT leads to greater increases in VO2 max but that MICT leads to reductions in body weight and higher heart rate.

A 2014 meta-analysis found that cardiorespiratory fitness, as measured by VO2 max, of individuals with lifestyle-induced chronic cardiovascular or metabolic diseases (including hypertension, obesity, heart failure, coronary artery disease, or metabolic syndrome) who have completed a HIIT exercise program, it was nearly double that of individuals who completed a MICT exercise program.

Metabolic benefits of HIIT

HIIT significantly reduces insulin resistance compared to low intensity training or inactive conditions and leads to a modest reduction in fasting glucose levels as well as an increase in weight loss compared to those who do not undergo a physical activity intervention.

Another study found that HIIT was more effective than continuous moderate-intensity training in reducing fasting insulin levels (31% decrease and 9% decrease).

HIIT and fat oxidation

A 2007 study looked at the physiological effects of HIIT on fat oxidation in moderately active women.

Study participants performed HIIT (defined as ten sets of 4' cycling repetitions with an intensity of 90% VO2max followed by 2' rest) on alternate days, for a period of 2 weeks. The study found that 7 HIIT sessions over a 2-week period improved body fat oxidation and skeletal muscle's ability to oxidize fat in moderately active women over 50 years of age. A 2010 systematic review of HIIT summarized HIIT results on fat loss and stated that HIIT may result in modest reductions in subcutaneous fat in young, healthy individuals, but greater reductions for overweight individuals.

HIIT and brain efficiency

A 2017 study looked at the effect of HIIT on cognitive performance in a group of 318 children. The authors show that HIIT is beneficial for cognitive control and working memory capacity compared to "a mixture of board games, computer games and quizzes" and that this effect is mediated by the brain-derived neurotrophic factor (BDNF). They conclude that the study suggests a promising alternative for improving cognition, through short and powerful exercise regimens.

Application

Since the concept of "high" intensity is related to a specific athletic ability, HIIT can be contextualized in different fields. Let's take a closer look at them.

Short-lasting HIIT, with an anaerobic and lactacid base

If referred to short-duration exercises, with an alactic and lactic anaerobic base, HIIT concerns both the maximal or submaximal expression of strength / rapidity / explosiveness, and resistance to strength / rapidity / explosiveness, both as close as possible to its limit. The limiting factor is always lactic acid. For example, in the first case you could perform 3 reps of flat bench press (rep) at 90% of 1RM, interspersed with a recovery of 6-7 ", for a number of series (sets) such as to achieve the inability to continue with the workout. In the second case, however, 25 burpees could be performed in 1'00", interspersed with a recovery of 20", for a series number (set) such as to achieve the inability to continue with the workout.

HIIT of medium and long duration, with anaerobic base complemented by anaerobic lactacid metabolism

If referred to medium and long duration exercises, with aerobic base completed by anaerobic lactate metabolism, it mainly concerns the expression of resistance to speed - rapid but cyclic movement, as in running, cycling, swimming, rowing, etc. resistance to medium and long duration strength - ability used in some particular sports, such as judo and brazilian jujitsu. In these cases, for example, the ground fight requires to maintain isometric contractions even for several minutes. For instance, in the first case - as in running - you could perform 5 rhythm variations in progression of 3', until reaching 90% of the maximal pulsations, alternating them with 1'30' 'of passive recovery which should guarantee a descent of the beats up to 135-145 per minute (bpm). In the second case instead, a circuit training could be set up with various isometric stations (isometric half squat, plank, side plank, isometric dip trust, etc.) lasting 3'00" each, interspersed with 1'30" of aerobic exercise, such as skipping, running, cycling or stepping.

Types of HIIT workouts

Peter Coe Protocol

It is a type of HIIT with short recovery periods used in the 1970s by coach Peter Coe. Inspired by the principles of Woldemar Gerschler and Swedish physiologist Per-Olof Åstrand, Coe established sessions that included repetitions of 200m fast running with only 30" of recovery.

Tabata Protocol

It is a HIIT version based on a 1996 study by Professor Izumi Tabata of the University of Ritsumeikan et al. It is based on 20" of ultra intense exercise (about 70% of VO2max) followed by 10" of rest, repeated continuously for 4 minutes (8 cycles).

Gibala Protocol

A 2010 study conducted by Professor Martin Gibala and his team at McMaster University in Canada is based on a HIIT structured as follows: 3' warm-up, 60" exercise at 95% VO2max, 75" rest, repeated for 8-12 cycles. The benefits are similar to what one would expect from a steady regimen at 50–70% VO2max five times a week.

Zuniga Protocol

Jorge Zuniga, assistant professor of exercise science at Creighton University, proposes a HIIT with 30" intervals at 90% of VO2 max, followed by 30" of rest.

Vollaard protocol

Dr. Niels Vollaard of the University of Stirling proposes a 10' training routine consisting of 6-10 maximum 30" sprints.

As you can see, there are different types of HIIT training that you can do. We recommend you to follow the classical Tabata protocol as it is one of the most effective there is. If you do not feel well during the exercise, please do not hesitate to stop, drink a glass of water and rest for a few minutes. The goal is to lose weight while staying healthy, never forget this!

<u>Chapter 3 - Before Fasting</u>

Now we have to point out some key concepts to follow in order to start your intermittent fasting diet with ease.

By following these ideas, you make sure to stay healthy and safe from the start. Once again, if you have questions, doubts or are not sure on how to approach this diet, follow the advice of your doctor.

Fasting means stopping food and drink for a specific period. People choose to fast to cleanse their digestive system, to lose weight, and in some cases, for spiritual or religious reasons.

Consult your doctor well in advance

During the fasting period, taking certain medications could be dangerous and have adverse effects on your health due to changes in blood chemistry. Fasting may not be suitable for people with particular health conditions, such as pregnancy, advanced cancer, low blood pressure, etc. Furthermore, your doctor will likely give you a urine or blood test before the fast begins.

Determine the type and duration of fasting you want to practice

Among the numerous ways of fasting we find water fasting, juice fasting, spiritual fasting, slimming fasting, etc. As we have seen, fasting can be extended from 1 to 30 days, depending on your specific goal. Research different fasting practices and choose the one that best suits your health condition and needs.

Be prepared for the changes that will take place in your body

As a result of the detoxification process, fasting can cause side effects such as diarrhea, exhaustion, fatigue, weakness, increased body odor, headache and more.

Consider taking a vacation from work or taking some time to relax throughout the day to limit the effects of fasting on your body.

It is important to know in advance the possible side effects caused by fasting, make sure that your research and your information are correct, detailed and comprehensive.

1 to 2 weeks before you start your fast, reduce your normal intake of addictive substances and break your eating habits. This procedure will reduce the potential withdrawal symptoms that you may experience during the fasting period. Addictive substances include alcohol, caffeinated beverages (such as tea, coffee, and carbonated drinks), cigarettes, and cigars.

Change your diet 1 to 2 weeks in advance
This means following these simple advice.

- Reduce your intake of chocolate and other foods that contain refined sugars and high percentages of fat.
- Reduce portion sizes during meals.
- Reduce the amount of meat and dairy you eat.
- Increase your intake of raw or cooked vegetables and fruit.
- In the days immediately before the fast begins, limit the amount of food you eat.

- Eat only raw fruits and vegetables, they will help cleanse and detox your body by preparing it for the fasting period.
- Drink only water and fresh, freshly prepared fruit and vegetable juices.

And most importantly, do not overthink what you are doing. We have stressed out how important it is to do things the right way, but we want to emphasize the fact that overthinking the process will not yield greater results. Just stay calm and collected during the entire process and you will start burning fat like crazy.

Nancy Johnson

Chapter 4 - What to Eat During an Intermittent Fasting Cycle

If the fasting component is important, when it comes to intermittent fasting nothing matters more than what you eat when you can actually consume your meals.

This is why we have decided to include this chapter that has the goal to give you the knowledge to craft healthy meals during your intermittent fasting cycle. As always, if in doubt, ask your doctor for nutritional advice.

Every single person has different food preferences and caloric and nutritional needs than others, but knowing the basic strategies for preparing a balanced meal can be of benefit to anyone. Balanced meals provide essential nutrients from various food groups, and can help you lose weight, improve cardiovascular function, and reduce the risks or side effects of many chronic conditions.

To make a balanced meal, half of the plate should be fruit and vegetables

You can eat fresh, frozen or canned fruit or vegetables, without adding other ingredients (such as sugar or salt).

The equivalent of a fresh fruit would be a glass of pure fruit juice or a handful of dried fruit. The equivalent of a serving of raw or cooked vegetables would be a glass of vegetable juice. Choose vegetables and fruits of various types: dark leafy vegetables, red and orange fruits, legumes (such as beans and peas), starchy vegetables and so on.

Eat whole grains, which should make up about a quarter of a balanced meal

At least half of the grains should be whole grain (not refined). Grains include food made from wheat, rice, oats, cornmeal, barley, and so on.

For example, bread, pasta, oatmeal, breakfast cereals, tortillas and semolina belong to the cereal group. Whole grains contain all the components of the grain. Examples include wholemeal flour, brown rice, oats, wholemeal corn flour and bulgur. Read the labels of the foods you want to buy to make sure they are whole and prefer them to refined products, such as white bread, white rice and so on.

Aim to eat a minimum of 85-120 grams of grains per day, remembering that the recommended amount for women over 50 is 170-230 grams. For example, you can eat 30 grams of pasta, rice or oatmeal, 1 slice of bread, and 1 cup of whole grain breakfast cereal.

Vary your protein sources to get more nutrients

Protein should make up about a quarter of the plate to make a balanced meal.

Eat both animal and plant proteins. The former include meat, poultry, fish and eggs, the latter legumes, nuts, seeds and soy. Choose several at each meal to get a good variety.

Aim for 140-170 grams of protein foods per day if you are a woman over 50 years of age. For example, you could eat 30 grams of lean meat, poultry or fish, 50 grams of cooked legumes or tofu.

Remember that proteins such as those contained in fish, nuts and seeds are also good sources of oils, equally essential for a balanced meal.

Add skim dairy products to get calcium and other nutrients found in cow's milk

Prefer the low-fat versions of these foods. Consume about 3 servings of dairy products per day. One serving is equivalent to a cup of milk (including soy) or a jar of yogurt. Eat 40g of plain cheese or 60g of processed cheese. Dairy products generally incorporate all foods derived from cow's milk. However, foods such as butter and cream cheese are usually not included in this group for nutritional reasons, as they are low in calcium.

If your intermittent fasting cycle ends with the breakfast, eat a full meal

To get your metabolism going, prepare your first meal of the day with foods from various food groups. Eat milk and cereals (you can choose the classic breakfast ones or make a soup), pieces of fresh and dried fruit or seeds. It is an easy to make and complete breakfast, in fact it has cereals, milk, fruit and proteins. Avoid sugary grains and fruits.

If you want a hot breakfast, make an omelet with 2 eggs or ½ cup of an egg substitute, 100 grams of vegetables (such as broccoli, peppers, and diced onions), and 30 grams of low-fat cheese.

Plan ahead for your meals

Once a week, buy all the ingredients you need for healthy cooking. Prepare several portions to eat throughout the week, or eat leftovers from dinner the next day for your next scheduled meal to save time but still have a proper intermittent fasting diet.

If you want to have a quick meal after you have finished your intermittent fasting cycle, make a sandwich with 2 slices of wholemeal bread, lettuce, onion, tomato, a slice of light cheese and a few slices of a cured meat of your choice. As a side dish, eat a salad with 2 tablespoons of dressing and a glass of pure fruit juice.

For a simple and balanced full meal, boil 150 grams of carrots, steam 180 grams of green beans, prepare 190 grams of brown rice and grill a pork chop. To drink, prefer water.

When planning meals and grocery shopping, cut back or eliminate prepackaged or pre-cooked foods, sodas, savory snacks, and desserts. If there are healthy and natural foods in the pantry, it is easier to eat well, without the temptation of ready-made industrial products.

Calculate your calorie needs

Determine how many calories to eat and how much to eat based on variables such as your age, weight and type of physical activity. Customize your meals accordingly. On many online websites it is possible to make specific calculations regarding your calorie needs.

Your calorie needs or ideal portions can change substantially or undergo changes due to various variables, such as the phase of the intermittent fasting program you find yourself in that moment.

Each meal should be balanced by calculating the right proportions of foods belonging to the various food groups. For example, don't eat large amounts of protein just to get more calories, or don't completely exclude a food group to reduce calorie intake.

Always consult a doctor

Make regular visits and consider any acute or chronic medical conditions you suffer from. Figure out which foods you should eat or avoid in your specific situation. Your condition may require you to change the portions of a typical balanced meal.

For example, people with diabetes may be advised to prefer whole grains to refined ones and to reduce their consumption of fruit or juice. Those with high cholesterol or heart disease should reduce their consumption of animal products and fatty foods. Those who need to lose weight can eat more vegetables and decrease the use of butter, oil, fat, sugar or salt in cooking.

Do not change your diet on the basis of general knowledge and clichés regarding the pathology you suffer from. To be sure that a modification is correct, you should always consult a doctor.

Make substitutions if you have an allergy or other dietary restrictions

If you have allergic reactions to certain types of foods, consider allergens. It may also be necessary to eliminate or substitute foods due to other health problems.

If you are lactose intolerant, include dairy products that are lactose-free or that contain a small amount of lactose, or replace cow's milk with a plant-based one, such as almond, soy, coconut, rice, and so on. Look for calcium-fortified foods and drinks or foods that are naturally high in calcium, such as sardines, tofu, tempeh, kale, and other leafy vegetables.

If you are a vegetarian or can consume products of animal origin in a limited way, prefer vegetable proteins such as legumes, nuts, seeds and soy in order not to have deficiencies.

While eliminating or limiting certain allergens, try to keep a balanced diet. Consult a dietician to explain how to meet your nutritional needs despite the restrictions and how to adapt your eating needs to an intermittent fasting regimen.

Weight Loss for Beginners

<u>Chapter 5 - Intermittent Fasting and the Right Mindset</u>

When starting an intermittent fasting cycle your mindset can make or break your ability to lose weight and burn fat.

In fact, it is your mind that will help you keep going when things will get difficult and uncomfortable. After all, if you decide to follow an intermittent fasting cycle you need to be prepared for things to get pretty wild when during the long fasting periods. By following these tips you make sure to have a strong mind that will support you in this transformative process.

The idea of starting a diet can be daunting, especially if you are not mentally prepared for such a change. When the mind is calm and prepared, sticking to a healthy eating plan is much easier. With the right preparation you will be able to effectively reach your goals and it will be less difficult not to fall into temptation along the way.

Be aware of recurring negative thoughts related to food

Often our diets fail because of our beliefs about food and eating. Try to become aware of your eating beliefs and make an effort to change your mindset.

We often think that on special occasions it is right to let yourself go a little. There's nothing wrong with eating a little more from time to time, but be honest with yourself about what you consider special occasions. When events like eating out, business lunches, office parties and other small events all become excuses for binging and breaking your intermittent fasting cycle, diet failure is just around the corner. So try to re-evaluate what can be considered a special occurrence.

Do you use food as a reward? Many think that after a long busy day it is normal to deserve to go out for dinner or eat a whole box of donuts. Look for alternative ways to reward yourself that don't include food. For example, pamper yourself with a long hot bath, buy yourself a new dress or go to the movies. There are many ways to reward yourself without resorting to food. Breaking your intermittent fasting routine should not be seen as a reward.

Dissociate food from certain activities

Food is closely linked to numerous daily rituals. Giving up sugar and fat may not be easy when we emotionally associate them with certain habits. Make a conscious effort to break through these dangerous associations.

Try to be aware of times when you overeat or make poor food choices, both in terms of food and what you drink. Do you indulge in Coke and popcorn every time you go to the cinema? Can't you say no to a few glasses of wine on evenings away from home? Can't you imagine a Saturday morning without coffee and donuts? If so, try to tear these associations apart.

You can do this by looking for alternatives. Do not think of food as a special treat, but consider it for what it truly is. It is just food. By making this powerful switch, you will see some immediate benefits, trust us on this.

Try changing associations by replacing unhealthy foods with healthier ones

For example, when spending the night out, play a board game instead of focusing on drinking. On Saturday mornings, when your intermittent fasting regimen allows you to eat, have breakfast with coffee, yoghurt and fresh fruit. If at the end of the day you tend to try to relax by eating, replace food with a good book or some music.

Start thinking about eating badly in terms of a habit rather than calories

In the long run, you will be more likely to stick to your diet by making a commitment to change negative behaviors rather than simply keeping calories in check. Try to be aware of when you eat bad foods and why you do it. Even if it's just half a cookie, ask yourself if you're indulging in it because you feel you've had a rough day. Do you tend to eat because you are hungry or because you feel bored? If you do this out of boredom, try to get rid of this bad habit. Even if you don't overdo the calories, always try to use common sense. Don't eat the wrong foods for the wrong reasons.

Ask for help and support

Changing is not easy and sometimes we are unable to do it alone. Ask for help from friends and family. Let them know that you are trying to lose weight with intermittent fasting and ask them to support you. Make sure they know they don't have to invite you to parties where cheap food and alcohol will be served. Also, ask to be able to let off steam with them at times when you feel particularly frustrated or tempted. Share your goals with all the people who live under your roof. Please keep tempting foods out of your sight, especially during fasting hours.

Set goals that are realistic

Many women tend to sabotage their diet by setting expectations too high. If you want to be able to stick to your plans, set achievable goals.

Remember that a balanced intermittent fasting diet allows you to lose about 1/2 to 1 pound per week, not more. If you intend to lose weight faster than this, be prepared to fail.

You should set cautious goals initially, so you will be more likely to achieve them and have the motivation to continue.

Keep a diary

If you want your intermittent fasting regimen to be successful you cannot avoid being accountable. Go out and buy a diary to accompany you along the entire journey. Record everything you eat daily and keep track of calories. A tangible account will force you to notice your bad habits and motivate you to develop new ones.

Plan your meals

Planning meals and snacks in advance will help you avoid giving in to temptation when fasting becomes difficult. In the days leading up to the intermittent fasting cycle, make a list of the healthy recipes you plan to make. Try to get ahead, for example by buying or cutting the necessary ingredients. If you want, you can also cook soups and vegetables to keep in the refrigerator, they will be very useful for the first week's meals.

Focus on concrete behaviors

If you limit yourself to analyzing your habits in abstract terms, it will not be easy to develop greater willpower. Reviewing your concrete actions will help you kickstart the transformation.

Make a list of the bad habits you intend to change. Start with small, gradual changes. Try to commit to abandoning an old behavior for a week, then continue slowly making new changes until you reach a positive and healthy lifestyle.

For example, decide that after work, instead of watching a show, you will walk for 40 minutes. Make a commitment to stick to your purpose for a week. Over the next few days, you can gradually increase the duration of the exercise, for example by increasing the distance or the duration of your walks.

Be trustworthy to yourself

On occasions when willpower is still not enough, work to get yourself back on track, even if it can mean having to be particularly hard on yourself. Doing so will help you understand that you are the only one who has the power to change your behaviors.

Acknowledge and respect your failures. Record them in your food diary. Take responsibility for failing.

Describe the reasons that led to your failure by highlighting your disappointment. For example, write something like "I ate dessert for dinner because I chose it and feel guilty after I did it". While these may seem harsh words, many find it helpful to make it clear that they have failed. You will feel motivated to make greater efforts to be able to change in the future. Trust us, this seems a hard method but it truly works incredibly well.

Consider giving in to temptation once a week

For some women, indulging in an "out of the box" weekly meal can be a great help in staying on track. A deprivation protracted for too long could shatter the entire intermittent fasting cycle. Sticking to a strict diet may seem more feasible when you know that at the end of the tunnel you can indulge in the coveted food. If you think it might help to control yourself, consider scheduling a reward meal at the end of the week or the fasting cycle.

While at the beginning you might think that you are strong enough not to need these tricks, we highly suggest to implement them from the beginning of your intermittent fasting regimen. This way, when things will get harder, because they will, you will already have the infrastructure and the right habits set up to help you deal with the difficulties of the moment.

Be gentle to yourself and respect your mind like you respect your body.

Weight Loss for Beginners

Chapter 6 - An Extreme Type of Fasting

In this chapter we would like to give you a quick overview of an extreme type of fasting that some women decide to use when they decide to lose weight. We do not know why, but there is this belief that it is possible to lose incredible amounts of fat by following what is known as water fasting.

While it is true that the numbers on the scale will go down rather quickly, it is also true that your health could be compromised if you decide to go down this path. While we advise you to avoid this extreme "diet", we know that some of you are interested in the topic. Therefore, we have decided to dedicate a chapter of this book to the best practices to do water fasting in a somewhat safe way. Again, please do not do this.

If you truly want to give water fasting a shot, consult a doctor before starting the practice.

There is no more detoxifying diet or a more demanding type of fasting than consuming water alone. It has no cost and can be used to lose weight, focus on the inner spiritual life and also to help the body excrete toxins. Short-term calorie restriction can help you live longer and healthier (if done correctly), but keep in mind that fasting can also be dangerous. Whatever your goal is, do it safely: take your time, work with a competent doctor, recognize the signs that you need to stop, and gradually return to normal eating.

Absolutely avoid fasting if you suffer from certain diseases

Some diseases can be aggravated with a restrictive diet and could lead to serious health consequences. Do not do a water fast if you have any of the following issues or health conditions, unless clearly approved by your doctor:

- Any eating disorder, such as anorexia or bulimia;

- Low blood sugar (hypoglycemia) or diabetes;

- Lack of enzymes;

- Kidney or liver disease in advanced stages;

- Alcoholism;

- Thyroid dysfunction;

- AIDS, tuberculosis or infectious diseases;

- Cancer in the advanced stage;

- Lupus;

- Vascular disease or poor circulation;

- Heart disease, including heart failure, arrhythmia (especially atrial fibrillation), previous heart attacks, valve problems, or cardiomyopathy;

- Alzheimer's disease or organic brain syndrome;

- Post-transplant complications;

- Paralysis;

- Pregnancy or breastfeeding;

- Pharmacological therapy that you cannot interrupt.

Decide how long you want to fast

Consider starting with just one day off from food and in any case not exceed three days if you are following the water fast alone, without the support of a doctor. Evidence has shown that a detox of as little as 1-3 days can offer health benefits; if you intend to go for multiple days, however, make sure you are supported and guided by a doctor, such as in the case of fasting retreats

It is arguably safer and offers greater health benefits to have periodic but short fasts, rather than just one for more than three days. Consider fasting on water for one day per week at the most.

Proceed when you are not very stressed

Schedule this detox when you are not under stress and when fasting does not interfere with normal daily activities; if possible, you shouldn't do this when you work. In fact, you should schedule it when you have time to rest physically and psychologically.

Prepare yourself mentally

The idea of fasting for several days may scare you; talk to your doctor, read books on the subject written by people with authority on this field and compare yourself with other individuals who have water fasted before. Live the experience as an adventure, but with cautious and respect for yourself.

Gradually progress towards fasting

You don't have to start suddenly and drastically, but slowly and progressively. First of all, start eliminating sugars, industrially processed foods, and caffeine from your diet for at least 2 to 3 days prior to this detox and eat mostly fruit and vegetables. Also consider reducing your meal portions for a few weeks before your fasting date. This can help prepare the body for what it is about to experience and mentally facilitate the transition to water fasting. Consider doing intermittent fasting to eventually end up consuming only water. Such a plan could last a month and follow this schedule.

- Week 1: don't eat breakfast;

- Week 2: skip both breakfast and lunch;

- Week 3: continue as in week 2 and reduce the portions of the dinner;

- Week 4: Water fasting begins.

Drink 9-13 glasses of water for a day

Generally speaking, women over 50 years of age should drink 13 8-ounce glasses of water or other liquids (about 3 liters or so) per day. You can stick to the dose during the water fast.

Make sure it's good quality water or drink filtered water at the very least.

Don't drink it all at once. Distribute your consumption throughout the day; prepare three bottles of one liter each day, in order to monitor their intake.

Do not exceed the recommended amount, as this could upset the balance of electrolytes and salts in the body, causing potential health problems.

Fight off hunger

If you complain of hunger attacks, overcome them by drinking a glass or two of water, then lie down and rest, the need for food usually goes away quickly; also try to distract yourself by reading or meditating.

Break the fast slowly and gradually

To break it up, start drinking an orange or lemon juice and then gradually add some solid food; for beginners, eat small amounts every two hours or so. Start with the foods that are easier to digest and continue gradually with the more demanding ones; depending on the length of your fast, you can spread this process over a day or more. Here is the order in which foods should be reintroduced in your diet after a water fast.

- Fruit juice;

- Vegetable juice;

- Raw fruit and green leafy vegetables;

- Yogurt;

- Vegetable soup and cooked vegetables;

- Cooked cereals and beans;

- Milk, dairy products and eggs,

- Meat, fish and poultry;

- Processed foods

Stick to a healthy diet after the water fast is complete

Fasting isn't very helpful if you go back to a high-fat, high-sugar diet. Plan a diet that includes lots of fruits, vegetables, whole grains and few unhealthy fats and refined sugars; exercise for half an hour a day, five days a week. Lead a healthy lifestyle to improve health, well-being and let water fasting be only a small part of this regimen.

Talk to your doctor before starting this process

If you are considering doing water fast, you must first consult a doctor. While it may offer health benefits for many people, others need to avoid it; so be sure to speak to an expert about your health condition and any treatments you are already taking to determine if it is safe for you to abstain from food. Your doctor is likely to decide to have a physical and blood test done before the start of the water fast.

If you are taking any medications, you should ask if you can continue taking them while fasting or if you need to change your dosage.

Fast under the supervision of an experienced practitioner

It is best to proceed under medical supervision, especially if you want to fast for more than three days or if you have any medical condition. Find a competent doctor in the field and let him guide you so that he can monitor your health during the process. Ask your family doctor if he can help you with this or if he recommends a qualified dietician or nutritionist who can follow you during the process.

Avoid vertigo

After two or three days of water fasting you may feel lightheaded when you get up too quickly; to prevent this from happening, try slowly standing up and breathing deeply before standing up. If you feel dizzy, sit or lie down immediately until you feel better; you can also try to put your head between the knees when you sit to feel more stable.

If the dizziness is severe enough to make you pass out, break your fast and go to the doctor immediately.

Distinguish normal from abnormal side effects

It is not uncommon to feel slightly dizzy, fainted, nauseated, or experience occasional arrhythmias when abstaining from food. However, you should stop practicing water fasting and seek medical help if you pass out, feel confused, have heart palpitations more than one time in a day or two, experience severe abdominal discomfort, headache or any other worrying symptom.

Get plenty of rest

You may find that you have less stamina and energy while water fasting; physical, emotional, sensory and psychological rest are an integral part of the process.

If you feel the need for a nap, go to bed; read something that lifts your mood, listen to your body and don't ask too much of it.

If you feel tired and dizzy, don't drive a vehicle and call your doctor.

Don't exercise intensely during this time

The energy level fluctuates from very low to very high, but even at the best of times you must avoid fatigue. Instead, try to follow some gentle and regenerating yoga sessions; it is a relaxing practice that stretches the muscles and allows you to do some light exercise.

Yoga and gentle stretching create well-being for some women, but may prove too vigorous for others; listen to your body and just do what you feel like. If your body asks for absolute rest, do not be afraid to give it to it.

Nancy Johnson

Chapter 7 - One Meal a Day (OMAD)

In this chapter we are going to discuss a particular type of intermittent fasting regimen. It is called the OMAD diet and the next few pages are going to tell you everything there is to know about it.

We are saturated with a culture of overeating and binge eating, and more and more people are exploring the concept that less can be more on many different levels. As can also be understood from the growing interest in a minimalist lifestyle, there is no doubt that we are trying to simplify our lives. So why not simplify our diet and eat once a day with the OMAD diet?

Similarly, several intermittent fasting (IF) and time-restricted feeding (TRF) protocols are on the wave of the trend. As we have seen, women are exploring different time windows in which they abstain from food or fast to improve health. Even though it is currently experiencing its best time in pop culture, fasting is nothing new. Fasting has been used throughout human history for spiritual and health reasons. From an ancestral perspective, always eating three or more times a day is not what humans have done for most of their existence, as they did not have constant access to the same quantities of food and were faced with regular periods of famine. Fasting is part of our DNA.

There are many ways to do intermittent fasting, from the simple 8-6 plan (eat between 8am and 6pm) to the fast-mimicking diet. The latter includes five days in which food can be ingested for the whole day and two with a maximum of 700 kcalories. A special way of doing intermittent fasting is the OMAD diet. OMAD sounds very exotic, but it literally means "One Meal a Day". An OMAD plan includes a fast of 23 hours a day and a 1 hour feeding window in which to eat. Normally this means waiting to eat until dinner, but in theory you can set a meal for one hour at any time of the day. Women over 50 usually practice OMAD to improve their health and energy, to lose weight, or both.

So is OMAD worth trying? Let's take a look at the things to consider.

The benefits of the OMAD diet

Given that OMAD is a more advanced type of intermittent fasting, there is a greater chance of achieving all the benefits that research has confirmed, such as:

- Higher levels of growth hormone, useful for increasing muscle and reducing fat;
- Lower levels of inflammation;
- Lower risk of diseases;
- Increased autophagy (cell recycling and repair).

Another key factor of intermittent fasting techniques such as OMAD is that natural ketosis is increased, which has benefits in terms of fat reduction and anti-inflammatory drugs. Since OMAD is longer fast, it tends to maximize these beneficial effects. Longer fasting windows give the body more time to push the benefits of fasting to the limit, while breaking the fast earlier tends to slow down these mechanisms.

Simplicity and convenience

OMAD fans love the fact that there is very little to plan with this fast (because there is only one meal to prepare!). The only plan that OMAD involves is that of the meal in which the fast is broken, to ensure that it has enough nutrients for the day.

Lower risk of diabetes

Given the characteristics of the OMAD diet, insulin levels will peak only once a day and for a short period of time (usually an hour), which means that the endocrine system is relaxed. This is in theory what connects intermittent fasting with both an improvement in cardiovascular capacity and with other diseases such as Type II diabetes or autoimmune diseases. This also leads to a lower risk of diabetes-related symptoms and other disorders directly related to diet and body metabolism.

It slows down aging

All types of intermittent fasting, but especially the OMAD diet, activate autophagy, with which the body cleanses itself of damaged cells, toxins, and waste. Autophagy also occurs in the neurons of the brain, which is why intermittent fasting has been shown to be beneficial in slowing down aging and in disorders such as Alzheimer's and Parkinson's.

Reduced calories

The OMAD diet can also make weight management easier given the natural calorie restriction. In fact, it becomes difficult to eat all the calories that you used to consume in a day in a single meal, but at the same time you still feel satisfied because that single meal is still satisfying in terms of taste, as you can cook almost whatever dish you like the most.

Chapter 8 - How to Eat Just One Meal a Day

In the previous chapter we have seen a specific type of intermittent fasting protocol that can help you maximize your weight loss chances. Some of you might be wondering how to actually apply this regimen in an effective and safe way.

In the next few pages, we are going to give you practical tips to fast for one full day, which is the skill you have to acquire in order to be successful with this "one meal a day" concept.

As we have seen, fasting means voluntarily avoiding eating for a given period of time. Some people fast to lose weight, others for religious or spiritual reasons. Whatever your reason for doing it, it is important to have a very strong motivation, because fasting is going against the natural instinct to eat. Having a clear purpose is essential to be able to achieve the goal. Before starting the fast, you should drink plenty of water, eat fruits and vegetables, and ensure your body a good night's sleep. By treating the body properly before, after and during the fast, you will be able to achieve greater mental clarity and burn more fat.

Ask yourself what you wish to learn from this experience - the answers will help you decide what the purpose of your fast day is. In all likelihood, you will achieve better results if you feel motivated to maintain self-control. You may want to fast for spiritual reasons, to achieve a state of mental clarity, or more simply to obtain physical benefits. If you are reading this book, we assume you are doing it because it is a great way to get in shape while being healthy.

Ask yourself questions and reflect on what motivates you and your goals. This is a simple trick that can help you a lot, especially when things get difficult. Besides losing weight, here are a couple of reason why you might be interesting in fasting for one full day.

- Fast to detoxify your body. Avoiding eating for a day will help your body more effectively excrete toxins, mucus, intestinal blockages, and other contaminants that damage your body.

- Fast to increase focus. Maybe you need to find a solution to a problem, understand a situation better, or get your intuitive and creative mind in motion. Fasting can help you achieve a greater state of mental clarity, which will allow you to analyze your problems more effectively.

Combine fasting with meditation, yoga or sensory deprivation practice to explore the depths of your mind. Use discipline and focus to escape the stimuli of hunger.

Often, when fasting for religious reasons, it is necessary to refrain from eating only until sunset. If you intend to follow the Islamic fasting rite, for example, you will have to stop eating twenty minutes before sunrise and can start again only twenty minutes after sunset. Fasting for 24 hours has become a very popular practice among those women who want to keep their body healthy and vigorous, especially among women who practice yoga on a daily basis.

It is best not to fast solely to lose weight. Even if this is an intermittent fasting book that teaches how this protocol can help you lose weight, we suggest you fast not just to lose a few pounds. There is more to that, as you might understand by now.

Fasting promotes the body's expulsion of toxins and can help you digest food more effectively, especially if practiced regularly. However, it is by no means certain that fasting will allow you to lose weight. Refraining from eating for a whole day and then bingeing on a large meal rich in carbohydrates means, for example, forcing the metabolism to reactivate in an extremely slow way. As a result, you will not burn more fat than you would have burned by eating normally.

If your only goal is to lose weight, try eating a breakfast that contains only very few calories instead of fasting for a full day. This light meal will activate the metabolism by causing the body to use up its fat reserves.

Consider fasting on juice only one day a week

With a liquid diet you can guarantee your body enough nutrients not to force it to use the sugar reserves stored in the liver and muscles. This way you will be able to detoxify the body without risking compromising muscle tissues.

Fasting allows you to start the body's self-healing process, with the advantage of improving your general health thanks to the break granted to the digestive system. Your organs will have time to take care of themselves. Fasting regularly helps you digest food more effectively, promotes greater mental clarity, increases physical and intellectual vigor, allows you to expel more toxins, improves vision and gives an intense feeling of general well-being.

Get ready for your full day of fasting

The day has almost arrived and your first 24 hours of fasting are right around the corner. It is important to get ready in the best possible way, in order to have a positive experience.

Here are a few practical tips you can follow to maximize your chance of having a smooth day.

The day before fasting, drink at least two liters of water

Water helps balance body fluids that promote blood circulation, saliva production, body temperature maintenance and digestion, as well as the absorption and distribution of nutrients. Be careful, this does not mean that you should drink an exaggerated amount of water immediately before starting the fast. In fact, the only result you would get would be to excrete it in the form of copious urine a few hours later. The right thing to do is to start drinking more in the 72 hours leading up to the fast.

Fruit juices, herbal teas, milk, energy drinks, and any other hydrating drink are helpful in preparing you to fast. Also try to eat foods rich in water, especially fruits and vegetables.

The day before your fast, eat healthy and nutritious foods

Absolutely avoid bingeing before you fast. It is much better to reduce portions than to increase them. If possible, eat mostly fruit and vegetables to balance your body. Eating food rich in water and nutrients can help your body prepare for fasting. Try to avoid baked foods, especially those that contain large amounts of salt or sugar.

During the 24 hours leading to the fast, it is also good to avoid all packaged foods notoriously rich in sugar. The human body is unable to function properly if it is fed mainly on sugars. Additionally, processed foods tend to stay in the digestive system longer, hindering the detoxification process that should come with fasting.

If you are diabetic, ask your doctor for advice on whether you can eat a lot of fruit without compromising your health.

Get a good night's sleep before you start fasting

The next day, the body will not be able to count on the caloric intake it is used to and will not be able to fight fatigue by eating foods that provide a lot of energy. By giving your body the necessary rest, you will help it function better during the day and you can benefit more from fasting.

We advise you to go to sleep an hour before you normally do. Our experience says that that extra hour will help you a lot in your mission.

The day of the fast

If you follow the tips we just gave you, you should have no problems during the fast. However, some women might find fasting a bit more challenging than others and need a bit more help to go through the process. The next few pages are full of interesting tricks you can apply to maximize your chances of success.

Please, always be aware that there is a difference between feeling challenged by the fast and feeling sick. If you do not feel well during the practice, just break the fast and eat something sweet to boost your sugar levels. If that does not help you feel better, call your doctor and ask for medical advice. Always have respect for yourself and your body.

Focus on the purpose of your fast
Direct your attention to the topics or questions you are looking for answers to. Focus on yourself, explore your intuitions, connect with your spirituality or simply let yourself be pervaded by discipline and self-control. If your goal is to detoxify your body, use it as an incentive to stay determined despite your hunger pangs.

If your fast allows you to drink only water, make sure you keep your body properly hydrated
Drink at least half a liter every two hours. Water fills the stomach, restores energy and dilutes digestive acids, which

give rise to the feeling of hunger. While drinking is important, try not to exceed the recommended doses so as not to risk getting sick.

Some religious practices, such as the Islamic fasting rite, prohibit drinking anything from sunrise until sunset. In this scenario, it is essential to hydrate the body abundantly before and after fasting.

Keep yourself busy

Inactivity and boredom can make you want to eat, so try to distract yourself by doing something exciting that isn't physically strenuous. Reading, writing, meditating, slowly practicing yoga, working on the computer, walking in nature, watching television, or driving short distances are all great ways to keep yourself busy while fasting. Avoid activities that require a lot of energy, such as lifting weights, going to the gym or running long distances. As we have seen in previous chapters, exercising at an intense level forces you to burn a lot of calories, making you too hungry.

Try not to think about food. It is best to stay away from the kitchen, supermarket or food images and scents.

Be persistent

If you feel like giving up, remind yourself of your reasons for fasting. Show your discipline and tell yourself that hunger won't last forever. If you can stay determined, the ultimate reward will be far more satisfying than a little food.

Towards the end of your fast, you are likely to feel tired and exhausted. At that moment you will have to appeal to all your tenacity. Take a nap if you can, or let yourself be distracted by pictures or videos. An engaging action movie or video game can be of great help in this situation.

Break your fast at the scheduled time

Start eating slowly, being very careful not to overdo the quantities. Cut servings in half. In fact, it's extremely important not to eat as much as you normally would because the digestive system has been paused and still can't handle a massive amount of food. Avoid meat, fish or cheese, it is much better to break the fast by eating some fruit, vegetables or soup. It is also important to drink water and fruit juices.

Remember not to eat and not to drink too much or too fast. Start with an apple and a glass of water, then wait about ten minutes. At this point, you can eat a small portion of the soup and drink a glass of orange juice.

Break the fast over a period of about 30-60 minutes. Eating a lot right away could cause severe abdominal pain and dysentery, putting your health at serious risk. Do things gently and gradually.

Weight Loss for Beginners

Chapter 9 - How to Fight the Urge to Eat

One of the most common difficulties women have when fasting is fighting the urge to eat. Oftentimes, this feeling is not associated with hunger itself but it has more to do with the habit of eating. In fact, most women are used to eating at least three meals a day and cutting back on this habit is not something easy to do.

While most books on intermittent fasting would tell you to just be strong and keep going, we know how difficult it can be not to break your fast when you are halfway through.

We want to do things differently and provide you with practical tips you can implement from the very beginning to fight the urge to eat.

Sometimes it can be helpful to learn how to control hunger. Being hungry all the time is frustrating and makes it difficult to maintain your ideal weight or stick to a diet plan. Many times it is not a question of real hunger or a physical need, but rather a manifestation of boredom. However, if your stomach is rumbling and you feel really hungry, there are a few things you can do to quickly reduce this feeling.

Do an inner analysis of your urge to eat

Whenever you feel hungry or have a desire to eat, pause for a few minutes and do a quick introspection. This way you can understand what is the best thing to do to deal with this feeling.

Many times you may feel hungry when in reality you are not really hungry. You may be bored, thirsty, agitated, stressed out, or just craving some tasty snack.

Since there are a number of reasons that could lead you to eat that are not strictly related to a physical need, it may be helpful to do this simple self-analysis first.

Take a few minutes to think about these questions and give yourself an honest answer.

Is your stomach "rumbling"? Do you have the impression that it is empty? When did you have your last meal or snack? Do you feel stressed, anxious or agitated? Are you bored?

Ask yourself these questions to understand if you really need to eat.

If yours is a real physical need for food, you may consider interrupting the fast to eat a simple snack or wait until it's time for the next meal. You can also do some little tricks to quench your hunger for a while.

If yours isn't true hunger, find some other activity to distract yourself until the craving for food subsides.

Drink water or tea

Many times you may feel hungry and want to nibble or eat something, but in reality you are just thirsty. Symptoms of hunger and thirst are similar, so they can be easily confused.

Water can help fill your stomach and keep you from experiencing hunger pangs. In fact, when the stomach contains water, it sends a satiety signal to the brain.

If your stomach "complains", drink two full glasses or consider always carrying a bottle of water with you and drinking throughout the day, sipping from time to time. This way, among other things, you avoid getting dehydrated.

Hot or lukewarm water makes you feel even more full than water at room temperature. The taste and the warmth can convey the same feeling of "satisfaction" as a meal. Hot coffee or tea are also good options. However, if you have to pay attention to avoid calories because you are fasting, choose sugar-free drinks.

Brush your teeth

It's a really quick way to curb hunger in just a few seconds. You will have a lot less desire to have a snack if your teeth are clean.

The toothpaste leaves an intense flavor in the mouth, which immediately takes away the desire to eat. Also, many foods no longer taste the same way right after brushing your teeth.

Always carry a travel toothbrush if you get hungry during a long day away from home.

Find a particularly exciting activity to do

If you think you are hungry but don't experience typical hunger symptoms, then your craving may be triggered by other factors.

It is very common to want to eat out of boredom. In this case, immediately take your mind off the food by doing some other activity, so as to distract your mind for a while and overcome the desire to eat.

Go for a brisk walk, talk to a friend, read a good book, do some housework, or surf the internet. One study found that when you play tetris you feel less craving for food, so it might be a good time to indulge in some gaming.

Grab a bubble gum or eat a candy
Some studies have found that these "tricks" help reduce the feeling of hunger immediately.

This technique is believed to be so effective because the sensation of chewing or sucking on a tasty product sends the signal to the brain that the body is satisfied.

Choose sugar-free gums and candies, as they have to have zero calories to avoid breaking the fast. These products typically contain no calories and are great for stopping hunger pangs when dieting.

Do not skip breakfast
While there are several ways to get hunger under control quickly, a good breakfast can help reduce the feeling of hunger throughout the day.

If you skip breakfast, you will likely feel a lot more hungry for the next few hours. In addition to this, a study has shown that not having this first meal leads to eating more calories in the rest of the day. If you never eat breakfast, your body tends to increase the insulin response, promoting weight gain.

Research has found that eating a breakfast high in fat, protein and carbohydrates reduces hunger throughout the day.

When you are following an intermittent fasting protocol, we suggest having a healthy breakfast and fast for the rest of your day, not the other way around.

Here are some suggestions for a breakfast that can help you in this regard.

- Scrambled eggs with low-fat cheese and wholemeal toast;
- wholemeal flour waffles with peanut butter and fruit;
- oatmeal with dried and fresh fruit.

Eat adequate amounts of proteins

As we have seen in previous chapters, these substances perform several important tasks in the body, but at the same time help you feel full longer than other nutrients.

Consuming protein also helps reduce cravings for sweet or high-fat foods.

Choose lean sources of protein (especially if you're particularly focused on weight loss) for each meal or snack. This way, you take them in adequate quantities for your needs, but you also feel satisfied and full throughout the day.

Among the various foods that provide lean protein you can consider: fish, poultry, lean beef, pork, eggs, low-fat dairy, legumes and tofu.

Make sure you eat protein foods within 30 minutes of exercising. Protein helps muscles absorb energy and develop. When following an intermittent fasting protocol, we advise you to exercise an hour after breaking your fast. In this way you have the time to eat something before your training session.

Choose foods that are rich in fiber

Several studies have found that people feel more satisfied and fuller by following a high-fiber diet than one that is deficient of this element.

There are several mechanisms that help induce the feeling of satiety with fibers. One of these is due to the fact that food that is rich in it has to be chewed a lot and takes longer to digest, thus increasing the sense of satiety. In addition, the fibers are voluminous, improving the feeling of fullness.

Vegetables, fruits, and whole grains are all high-fiber foods that typically leave you with a longer lasting sense of satisfaction than other foods.

Salads and vegetable soups are particularly valuable in this regard, as they are high in fiber and low in calories.

Another good thing about fiber is that it helps regulate blood sugar levels, keeping hunger pangs in check.

Satisfy your food cravings in a healthy way

There are probably many occasions when you are not really hungry, but want to have a snack or treat. A few concessions from time to time is fine, especially if you choose to satisfy this "craving" in a healthy way. However, do not make it a habit to break your fast when you are not supposed to. Remember, creating a healthy intermittent fasting protocol means having the discipline to follow your plan.

There are several healthy alternatives to candy and salty, crunchy foods to calm the craving for food. Choose your snack wisely.

If you are craving for dessert, eat some fruit. An apple or orange provides fiber and vitamins, as well as some sugar to satisfy the need for sweetness.

If you feel craving for something more salty and crunchy, grab a small serving of salted nuts. Eat raw vegetables with hummus to satisfy the need for salty and crunchy.

However, once again we recommend you break the fast only if the urge to eat is too hard to fight. We encourage you to push yourself a bit as intermittent fasting can be a great mind exercise as well.

Chapter 10 - How to Understand If You Are Truly Hungry or Not

During previous chapters we have mentioned different times how important it is to understand when you are too hungry to continue the fast and when you are just bored and have food cravings.

However, most women are so out of touch with their bodies that cannot properly distinguish these two very different situations. They have been conditioned over the years that each time their belly says something, it is important to answer by eating something. The following pages will give you a better understanding of the processes that you can put in place to understand if you are truly hungry or if you are just not accustomed to the feeling of intermittent fasting. Having a good grasp of this difference allows you to make better decisions and helps you stick to the protocol.

By practicing these tricks on a regular basis, you will develop your instinct and know when it is time to push it through and when it is better to have a snack.

It can be quite difficult to distinguish physical from emotional hunger. This is especially true if you are not very familiar with recognizing the signals your body is sending you. Physical hunger typically comes on gradually and subsides after eating a meal. However, some women often tend to eat even when they don't really need to eat. In this case, it is emotional hunger that leads to eating when you are in certain psychological states: stress, boredom, anxiety, happiness or even depression. Therefore, understanding hunger and knowing how it affects the body can help distinguish between a symptom of a physiological need and an emotional problem. This chapter is intended to give you some tips to learn about your body, hunger levels, and how to avoid the temptation to eat when in reality it is not yet time to feed.

Rank your hunger level on a scale of 1 to 10

This method can help you figure out what to do. It should give you an idea on whether to eat a snack and break the fast or wait until the next scheduled meal. Try to establish hunger from level 1 (almost faint from hunger) to level 10 (completely full, almost nauseous).

If your hunger level is around 3 or 4, it may be time to eat even if your intermittent fasting protocol says not to do it. If your next meal isn't scheduled within a couple of hours, have a snack. If, on the other hand, you are expected to eat within an hour or so, try to hold on until you sit down at the table.

In theory, you shouldn't go to extremes: neither go hungry at level 1, nor overdo it and eat until level 10. Try to stick to the 4-7 values.

It is normal and predictable to feel hungry before a meal and even just before going to sleep in the evening.

Take the apple test

This is a simple test that can help you figure out if you are having a physical or emotional hunger attack. Typically, psychological hunger is the need and desire to eat something from a particular food group (such as carbohydrates) or a specific food (such as chocolate cake). Physical hunger, on the other hand, is satisfied with a wide variety of foods.

Ask yourself if you want to eat a snack even if it was an apple, a raw carrot or a salad.

If so, eat an apple (another fruit or vegetable) or another healthy, planned snack that really satisfies your physical hunger.

If not, you probably need to satisfy an emotional hunger and not a physical hunger.

If you have determined that it is psychological hunger, this is the right time to go for a walk or take a 10-minute break and reflect on the reason for your upset.

Observe yourself

Before eating any meal or snack, take a minute or two to analyze yourself internally. By doing this, you can understand your true level of hunger and desire to eat.

Evaluate various aspects such as the level of hunger. Do you feel undernourished? Are you full instead? Do you feel satisfied?

Take note of the physical signs of hunger. Your stomach may "grumble", you may feel empty or feel hunger cramps, if it is a real need to eat.

If you feel the desire to eat something without a real physical need, analyze your emotional state. Are you bored? Have you had a stressful day at work? Do you feel tired or exhausted?

Many times these moods induce a feeling of "hunger" when in reality it is not a real physical need to eat food.

Drink enough water

Aim to drink adequate amounts of fluids each day. Usually, it is recommended to drink about 8 glasses or almost 2 liters of water. This is just a general recommendation. In fact, you could drink a little more or a little less. Proper hydration helps you lose weight, but it's also important for managing hunger levels throughout the day.

If you are thirsty or a little dehydrated, you may experience a feeling of hunger. If you don't drink properly every day, dehydration can trigger hunger, which can cause you to eat more food or more often than you need to.

Keep a bottle of water on hand at all times and pay attention to how much you drink each day. Also, try to drink just before a meal to calm hunger and reduce food intake.

Wait 10 to 15 minutes and see what happens

Emotional hunger can come on suddenly, but it can disappear just as quickly, unlike the physical need to eat. If you take 10-15 minutes of distraction from the situation you are experiencing, you may find that your food cravings and emotional urge to eat are reduced and you are able to control them much more easily.

By waiting a few minutes, the craving for food does not completely disappear, but it subsides enough to be able to overcome it with willpower.

Try telling yourself that during this time you can re-evaluate your ideas about eating some specific food or snack. Engage in another activity, but go back to considering breaking the fast if the need is still there.

Empty the kitchen

If you have a fridge or pantry full of unhealthy foods that tempt you, it can be easier to give in to emotional hunger. If you know that you can easily have a packet of crackers or a bag of chips when you are bored or stressed, do not keep these foods at home, so as not to be tempted when you are overwhelmed by these feelings; by doing so, you can eat less if you are not really hungry.

Take an hour or two to scan the kitchen. Check the pantry, fridge, freezer, and cupboards at home where you keep food. Put all the foods and snacks that make you want to eat on the table and examine them to decide which ones to keep and which ones to discard.

Donate any still packaged items to the food counter or church if you don't want to throw them in the trash.

Make a promise to yourself not to buy tempting but unhealthy snacks anymore, so that your kitchen and home are healthy environments.

Get away from food

Sometimes, the very fact of being in the same room as your favorite foods or some food you crave to eat makes it harder to ignore the urge to fill your belly. If you are in a place in your home or office that increases your desire to eat, get away. Take the time and space to clear your mind of the need for some "rewarding treats".

Take a walk for 15 minutes if you can. Distract your mind and bring attention to other thoughts that are not related to nutrition.

Sometimes, some people feel the urge to have some nighttime snacks. Instead of staying awake, go to bed. In this way, you stay away from the kitchen and aren't tempted to unwittingly eat in front of the TV. If you are not tired, read a good book or magazine until you are sleepy enough to fall asleep.

Make a list of the things you can do instead of eating

This "trick" can distract your mind from food cravings and help you manage emotional hunger. Make a quick list of activities that you enjoy or that distract you enough to take your thoughts away from food. Here are some ideas-

- Clean the cupboards or rearrange the junk drawer;

- Take a walk;

- Engage in your favorite hobby;

- Read a book or magazine;

- Play a game.

Eat a small portion of the food you just can't resist

Sometimes, the need or desire to eat can overwhelm you uncontrollably. Even if you get distracted and try to reduce the craving for food, it can be very intense. If that is the case, some experts recommend consuming a small, controlled portion of that food you crave to eat.

By limiting yourself to a small portion, you can reduce your food cravings, but at the same time allow yourself the pleasure of eating something tasty.

Make sure it's a very small portion. Read the nutrition label and measure the appropriate amount, put the rest away and slowly enjoy your dose so you can enjoy all the flavor.

Please, note that this practice still counts as breaking the fast. So do not use it unless the craving is unbearable.

Keep a diary

It is a great tool for raising awareness and managing emotional hunger. You can use it to understand where and when you eat, which types of foods give you the most comfort, and which ones you want to eat most often.

Purchase a food diary or download a smartphone app. Monitor as many days as possible - both during the week and on the weekend. Many people eat differently on weekends, so it's important to take note of both situations.

Also take into account any feelings or moods you experience when you eat. This can help you learn more about the emotions that cause you to eat certain foods.

Talk to a qualified dietician or behavioral therapist

These health professionals can help you manage emotional hunger. If you are having trouble keeping your appetite in check or you see that it is putting your health at risk, it is a wise idea to keep in touch with a doctor.

The dietician is an experienced nutritionist who can help you understand emotional hunger, explain true physical hunger to you, and can point you to alternative food options.

The behavioral therapist will help you understand why you are feeling emotional hunger and can give you some tips to change your reactions and behavior in the face of certain triggers.

Find a support group

Regardless of your health goal, a support group plays an important role in achieving long-term positive results. This is even more true when hunger is emotional. Having this kind of support when you're feeling sad or stressed can help you lift your mood without the need for food.

Whether it's your spouse, family, friends, or coworkers, a support group can motivate and encourage you as you progress.

Also look for an online support group or people who gather for this purpose in your city. Email new friends who share your long-term goals and tell them about your intermittent fasting protocol.

Having someone by your side will make all the difference in the world.

Nancy Johnson

Conclusion

We would like to thank you for making it to the end of this book. We have done our best to ensure that every information contained is useful and helps you in your weight loss journey.

We know how frustrating it could be to start an intermittent fasting protocol and feeling discouraged by the fact that results do not appear immediately. As we repeated throughout the book, the goal of intermittent fasting is to create a healthy lifestyle that can support you over the years, not just give you a rapid decrease in weight.

By following the tips shared in this book, you will certainly burn fat, lose weight and feel much better. However, as we do not know you in person, our final recommendation can only be the following one.

Before starting an intermittent fasting protocol talk to your doctor and find out whether intermittent fasting could be a good idea for you or not. Remember, never sacrifice your health to fit into that new skirt you just got.

To your success!

Lightning Source UK Ltd.
Milton Keynes UK
UKHW012122120521
383626UK00001B/25